INTERVENTIONAL CARDIOLOGY CLINICS

www.interventional.theclinics.com

Editor-in-Chief

MATTHEW J. PRICE

Transcatheter Mitral Valve Repair and Replacement

July 2019 • Volume 8 • Number 3

ELSEVIER

1600 John F. Kennedy Boulevard • Suite 1800 • Philadelphia, Pennsylvania, 19103-2899

http://www.theclinics.com

INTERVENTIONAL CARDIOLOGY CLINICS Volume 8, Number 3
July 2019 ISSN 2211-7458, ISBN-13: 978-0-323-67880-3

Editor: Lauren Boyle
Developmental Editor: Donald Mumford

Interventional Cardiology Clinics (ISSN 2211-7458) is published quarterly by Elsevier Inc., 360 Park Avenue South, New York, NY 10010-1710. Months of issue are January, April, July, and October. Subscription prices are USD 203 per year for US individuals, USD 474 for US institutions, USD 100 per year for US students, USD 204 per year for Canadian individuals, USD 565 for Canadian institutions, USD 150 per year for Canadian students, USD 296 per year for international individuals, USD 565 for international institutions, and USD 150 per year for international students. To receive student/resident rate, orders must be accompanied by name of affiliated institution, date of term, and the *signature* of program/residency coordinator on institution letterhead. Orders will be billed at individual rate until proof of status is received. Foreign air speed delivery is included in all *Clinics* subscription prices. All prices are subject to change without notice. **POSTMASTER:** Send address changes to *Interventional Cardiology Clinics*, Elsevier Health Sciences Division, Subscription Customer Service, 3251 Riverport Lane, Maryland Heights, MO 63043. **Customer Service: Telephone: 1-800-654-2452** (U.S. and Canada); **1-314-447-8871** (outside U.S. and Canada). **Fax: 1-314-447-8029. E-mail: journalscustomerservice-usa@elsevier.com (for print support); journalsonlinesupport-usa@elsevier.com (for online support).**

Reprints. For copies of 100 or more of articles in this publication, please contact the Commercial Reprints Department, Elsevier Inc., 360 Park Avenue South, New York, NY 10010-1710. Tel.: 212-633-3874; Fax: 212-633-3820; E-mail: reprints@elsevier.com.

CONTRIBUTORS

EDITOR-IN-CHIEF

MATTHEW J. PRICE, MD
Director, Cardiac Catheterization Laboratory,
Division of Cardiovascular Diseases,
Scripps Clinic, La Jolla, California, USA

AUTHORS

LUCIA ALVAREZ, MD
Fellow, Division of Cardiology, Emory
University, Atlanta, Georgia, USA

ANITA W. ASGAR, MD, MSc
Associate Professor, Department of Medicine,
Montreal Heart Institute, Faculté de
médecine, Université de Montréal, Montréal,
Québec, Canada

VASILIS BABALIAROS, MD
Professor, Division of Cardiology,
Emory University, Atlanta, Georgia,
USA

JEREMY BEN-SHOSHAN, MD
Department of Medicine, Montreal
Heart Institute, Faculté de médecine,
Université de Montréal, Montréal, Québec,
Canada

STEVEN F. BOLLING, MD
Department of Cardiac Surgery, University of
Michigan Health System, Ann Arbor,
Michigan, USA

WALTER D. BOYD, MD
Division of Cardiothoracic Surgery,
University of California, Davis Medical
Center, Sacramento, California, USA

ISIDA BYKU, MD
Fellow, Division of Cardiology, Emory
University, Atlanta, Georgia,
USA

THIERRY CARREL, MD
Department of Cardiovascular Surgery, Bern
University Hospital, Bern, Switzerland

CHARLES J. DAVIDSON, MD
Chief, Division of Cardiology, Northwestern
University Feinberg School of Medicine,
Chicago, Illinois, USA

DHAVAL DESAI, MD
Division of Cardiovascular Diseases,
Scripps Clinic, La Jolla, California,
USA

MARIO GÖSSL, MD, PhD
Valve Science Center, Minneapolis
Heart Institute Foundation, Abbott
Northwestern Hospital, Minneapolis,
Minnesota, USA

ISAAC GEORGE, MD
Department of Cardiovascular Surgery,
Bern University Hospital, Bern,
Switzerland

PATRICK GLEASON, MD
Assistant Professor, Division of
Cardiology, Emory University, Atlanta,
Georgia, USA

ADAM GREENBAUM, MD
Associate Professor, Division of
Cardiology, Emory University, Atlanta,
Georgia, USA

CHETAN HUDED, MD, MSc
Interventional Cardiology Fellow, Cleveland
Clinic Heart and Vascular Institute, Cleveland,
Ohio, USA

NORIHIKO KAMIOKA, MD
Fellow, Division of Cardiology,
Emory University, Atlanta, Georgia,
USA

SAMIR KAPADIA, MD
Section Head of Interventional Cardiology,
Director of Sones Cardiac Catheterization
Laboratory, Cleveland Clinic Heart and
Vascular Institute, Cleveland, Ohio,
USA

MOHAMMAD KASSAR, MD
Department of Cardiology, Bern University
Hospital, Bern, Switzerland

OMAR K. KHALIQUE, MD
Structural Heart and Valve Center,
Division of Cardiology, NewYork-Presbyterian
Hospital/Columbia University Medical
Center, New York City, New York,
USA

JAFFAR M. KHAN, BM, BCh
Fellow, Division of Cardiology, Washington
Hospital Center, Washington, DC,
USA

OLGA N. KISLITSINA, MD, PhD
Research Associate Professor, Cardiology,
Northwestern University Feinberg School of
Medicine, Chicago, Illinois, USA

ROBERT LEDERMAN, MD
Interventional Cardiologist, Cardiovascular
Branch, Division of Intramural Research,
National Heart, Lung, and Blood Institute,
National Institutes of Health, Bethesda,
Maryland, USA

JOHN LISKO, MD, MPH
Fellow, Division of Cardiology,
Emory University, Atlanta, Georgia,
USA

RAJ MAKKAR, MD
Cedars-Sinai Smidt Heart Institute, Los
Angeles, California, USA

PATRICK M. McCARTHY, MD
Executive Director of the Bluhm
Cardiovascular Institute, Chief,
Division of Cardiac Surgery, Heller-Sacks
Professor of Surgery, Northwestern
University Feinberg School of Medicine,
Northwestern University, Chicago, Illinois,
USA

SUKIT CHRIS MALAISRIE, MD
Associate Professor of Surgery, Division of
Cardiac Surgery, Northwestern University
Feinberg School of Medicine, Chicago, Illinois,
USA

HIROKI NIIKURA, MD
Valve Science Center, Minneapolis
Heart Institute Foundation, Abbott
Northwestern Hospital, Minneapolis,
Minnesota, USA

THOMAS PILGRIM, MD
Department of Cardiology, Bern University
Hospital, Bern, Switzerland

FABIEN PRAZ, MD
Department of Cardiology, Bern
University Hospital, Bern, Switzerland;
Department of Cardiothoracic
Surgery, NewYork-Presbyterian
Hospital/Columbia University
Medical Center, New York City,
New York, USA

MATTHEW J. PRICE, MD
Director, Cardiac Catheterization Laboratory,
Division of Cardiovascular Diseases,
Scripps Clinic, La Jolla, California,
USA

DAVID REINEKE, MD
Department of Cardiovascular
Surgery, Bern University Hospital,
Bern, Switzerland

JASON H. ROGERS, MD
Division of Cardiovascular Medicine,
University of California, Davis Medical
Center, Sacramento, California,
USA

TOBY ROGERS, PhD, BM, BCh
Interventional Cardiologist, Cardiovascular
Branch, Division of Intramural Research,
National Heart, Lung, and Blood
Institute, National Institutes of
Health, Bethesda, Maryland,
USA

THOMAS W. SMITH, MD
Division of Cardiovascular Medicine,
University of California, Davis Medical
Center, Sacramento, California,
USA

PAUL SORAJJA, MD
Roger L. and Lynn C. Headrick Chair, Valve
Science Center, Minneapolis Heart Institute
Foundation, Abbott Northwestern Hospital,
Minneapolis, Minnesota, USA

DEE DEE WANG, MD
Director of Structural Heart Imaging, Center
for Structural Heart Disease, Henry Ford
Health System, Detroit, Michigan, USA

STEPHAN WINDECKER, MD
Department of Cardiology, Bern
University Hospital, Bern,
Switzerland

SUNG-HAN YOON, MD
Cedars-Sinai Smidt Heart
Institute, Los Angeles, California,
USA

CONTENTS

Treatment of Functional Mitral Regurgitation with Transcatheter Edge-to-Edge Repair
Chetan Huded and Samir Kapadia

Mitral valve regurgitation is a common valvular lesion affecting approximately 1 in 10 older adults, and it can be broadly categorized as degenerative or functional in etiology. Although transcatheter mitral valve repair with the MitraClip is currently approved for commercial treatment of severe degenerative mitral regurgitation, its role in patients with functional mitral regurgitation is evolving. Two recent pivotal trials have evaluated the effectiveness of the MitraClip device in those with severe functional mitral regurgitation. We review the concepts of edge-to-edge mitral valve repair and evidence regarding transcatheter edge-to-edge repair with MitraClip in patients with functional mitral regurgitation.

Transcatheter Edge-to-Edge Repair for Primary (Degenerative) Mitral Regurgitation: Registries and Trials
Dhaval Desai and Matthew J. Price

The MitraClip is the only approved transcatheter edge-to-edge repair device that is commercially available for the treatment of severe, symptomatic, primary (degenerative) mitral regurgitation in patients deemed to be at prohibitive risk by a heart team. Transcatheter edge-to-edge repair can be safely performed with a low rate of periprocedural adverse events despite a predominantly elderly patient population with multiple comorbidities. Transcatheter edge-to-edge repair is associated with improvement in mitral regurgitation severity; left ventricular dimensions and remodeling; heart failure rehospitalizations; and, in high-risk groups, an improvement in survival compared with medical therapy.

Transcatheter Mitral Valve Direct Annuloplasty with the Millipede IRIS Ring
Jason H. Rogers, Walter D. Boyd, Thomas W. Smith, and Steven F. Bolling

Mitral valve ring annuloplasty is a surgical gold standard and is used routinely during surgical mitral valve repair of primary or secondary mitral regurgitation. The Millipede IRIS annuloplasty ring is the first transcatheter, transfemoral, transseptal, semirigid, complete annuloplasty ring to be delivered to the mitral valve annulus. Initial results in humans demonstrate that the Millipede IRIS ring is safe, and can effectively reduce the mitral annular diameter leading to a clinically significant reduction or elimination of mitral regurgitation.

Left Ventricular Outflow Tract Obstruction: A Potential Obstacle for Transcatheter Mitral Valve Therapy
Jeremy Ben-Shoshan, Dee Dee Wang, and Anita W. Asgar

Transcatheter mitral valve replacement is the focus of much enthusiasm as the future of therapy for mitral valve disease. Despite technological advances, left ventricular outflow tract (LVOT) obstruction from the valve prosthesis remains an important issue. In this review the authors discuss the pathophysiology of LVOT obstruction in both the surgical and transcatheter experience, imaging evaluation preprocedure, outcomes to date, and therapeutic options.

Transcatheter mitral valve replacement (TMVR) is a promising strategy for patients with mitral valve disease and no surgical options. Left ventricular outflow tract (LVOT) obstruction is a life-threatening complication of TMVR. Although there are no commercially available devices to prevent LVOT obstruction, the risk of it can be reduced by careful preprocedure planning and the use of novel modifications to commercially available devices. This article summarizes current techniques to prevent LVOT obstruction with an emphasis on electrosurgical strategies.

Transcatheter mitral valve replacement with the Intrepid device is intended for patients who need mitral valve replacement and who are at an increased risk for conventional surgery. The early published results of the early feasibility trial are reviewed as well as device design and the implant procedure. The Apollo trial is reviewed: a randomized trial of the Intrepid device versus conventional surgery including a single arm study for inoperable patients. The mitral valve structure, pathophysiology, and postimplant physiology pose unique hurdles for any transcatheter implant.

Mitral regurgitation is the most commonly occurring valvular heart disease in developed countries. Transcatheter mitral valve replacement (TMVR) has emerged as a novel potential therapy for patients with severe mitral valve disease who are unsuitable candidates for conventional surgery or transcatheter edge-to-edge mitral repair. TMVR with the Tendyne prosthesis has shown potential at short-term follow-up to be an effective and safe treatment alternative for high-risk patients with severe mitral valve disease.

Mitral annular calcification (MAC) is a fibrous, degenerative calcification of the mitral valve. It is associated with endocarditis, coronary artery disease, valvular heart disease, and congestive heart failure. Patients with severe MAC associated with mitral valve disease are considered poor candidates for traditional surgery. The current available outcomes data of transcatheter mitral valve replacement (TMVR) in severe MAC were limited by high rates of serious complications and subsequent high short-term and midterm mortality. This review article describes the procedural complications, clinical outcomes, and optimal patient selection for TMVR in patients with severe MAC.

Surgical mitral valve replacement in patients with severe annular calcification is a challenge for the cardiac surgeon. Surgical transatrial implantation of a transcatheter heart valve is an alternative for selected patients, in particular those at risk for obstruction of the left ventricular outflow tract or valve embolization. Herein, we review patient selection, surgical technique, and early outcomes after this novel hybrid procedure.

TRANSCATHETER MITRAL VALVE REPAIR AND REPLACEMENT

FORTHCOMING ISSUES

October 2019
Hot Topics in Interventional Cardiology
Matthew J. Price, *Editor*

January 2020
Transradial Angiography and Intervention
Binita Shah, *Editor*

RECENT ISSUES

April 2019
Updates in Percutaneous Coronary Intervention
Matthew J. Price, *Editor*

January 2019
Congenital Heart Disease Intervention
Daniel S. Levi, *Editor*

October 2018
Transcatheter Aortic Valve Replacement
Susheel K. Kodali, *Editor*

RELATED SERIES

Cardiology Clinics
Cardiac Electrophysiology Clinics
Heart Failure Clinics

THE CLINICS ARE NOW AVAILABLE ONLINE!

Access your subscription at:
www.theclinics.com

PREFACE

Transcatheter Mitral Valve Repair and Replacement: New Standards of Care and New Horizons for Therapy

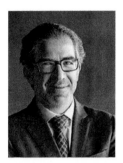

Matthew J. Price, MD
Editor

After many years of being considered the "next big thing," transcatheter approaches to mitral valve disease have reached a turning point. Transcatheter edge-to-edge repair, approved in the United States since the spring of 2013 and performed in more than 75,000 patients to date worldwide, has become an accepted therapy for patients with primary (degenerative) mitral regurgitation who are at prohibitive risk for open repair or replacement. In the setting of functional mitral regurgitation, where surgical therapy has not been proven nor embraced, the prospective, randomized COAPT trial recently demonstrated that transcatheter edge-to-edge repair, when combined with maximally tolerated guideline-directed medical therapy, reduces recurrent heart failure hospitalization and decreases mortality compared with optimal guideline-directed medical therapy alone. These findings show that in patients with mitral regurgitation associated with left ventricular dysfunction, the regurgitation itself, and not only the ventricle, is a driver of poor clinical outcomes. However, due to anatomic constraints, not all mitral regurgitation can be addressed by the current transcatheter edge-to-edge repair technology, and improvements in mitral regurgitation reduction with transcatheter repair could in theory further improve long-term outcomes. Transcatheter mitral annuloplasty and transcatheter mitral valve replacement represent the next horizons for therapy. The development of transcatheter mitral valve replacement has been challenging due to particular anatomic hurdles and device profiles, but the pivotal randomized trials have recently commenced for two such valve therapies. Finally, novel approaches to treat mitral stenosis and regurgitation in patients with severe mitral annular calcification are being

Intervent Cardiol Clin 8 (2019) xi–xii
https://doi.org/10.1016/j.iccl.2019.04.001
2211-7458/19/© 2019 Published by Elsevier Inc.

reported, which it is hoped will address this difficult-to-treat and highly comorbid patient cohort.

The number of subspecialty journals has expanded greatly in the past decade, which makes it hard for the busy Interventional Cardiologist to keep up with the latest developments and data in our field. My goal as Editor-in-Chief of *Interventional Cardiology Clinics* has been to distill this information by inviting key thought leaders and the investigators involved in the seminal studies to provide up-to-date reviews of their work. I believe this current issue has accomplished, and exceeded, this task.

Matthew J. Price, MD
Division of Cardiovascular Diseases
Scripps Clinic
9898 Genesee Avenue
AMP-200
La Jolla, CA 92037, USA

E-mail address:
price.matthew@scrippshealth.org

Treatment of Functional Mitral Regurgitation with Transcatheter Edge-to-Edge Repair

Chetan Huded, MD, MSc, Samir Kapadia, MD*

KEYWORDS

- Mitral regurgitation • Mitral insufficiency • Mitral valve disease • Mitraclip
- Transcatheter mitral valve repair

KEY POINTS

- Edge-to-edge mitral valve repair has been performed historically with a surgical procedure and more recently with a catheter-based device (MitraClip).
- Transcatheter edge-to-edge mitral valve repair with MitraClip has been approved for commercial use in Europe since 2008 and for use in degenerative mitral regurgitation among inoperable patients in the United States since 2013.
- The MitraClip recently gained FDA approval for commercial use in functional mitral regurgitation in the United States based on two recent pivotal clinical trials.
- The MITRA-FR and COAPT trials provided conflicting results on the safety and effectiveness of transcatheter edge-to-edge mitral valve repair with MitraClip in functional mitral regurgitation. Important differences in patient population, study administration and procedural success may contribute to the differing results observed in these 2 trials.

INTRODUCTION

Mitral regurgitation (MR) is the most common form of valvular heart disease. The prevalence of MR increases significantly with age, and the prevalence in patients ≥75 years old is approximately 1 in 10.[1] Mitral regurgitation can be broadly categorized as degenerative MR (DMR) or functional MR (FMR) based on the mechanism of mitral valve insufficiency (Table 1). Degenerative mitral regurgitation, also referred to as primary MR, includes mitral valve insufficiency related to anatomic abnormalities of the mitral valve leaflet or subvalvular apparatus. Functional mitral regurgitation, also referred to as secondary MR, refers to mitral valve insufficiency secondary to abnormalities of the left ventricle or left atrium, which distort the coaptation of the valve leaflets. Functional mitral regurgitation is the consequence of underlying structural heart disease of various etiologies. Successful management of FMR requires a multifaceted approach including treatment of the underlying cardiomyopathy, volume management, afterload reduction, and cardiac resynchronization therapy in eligible patients (Fig. 1). In those patients with severe FMR and lifestyle limiting heart failure symptoms despite the aforementioned therapies, mitral valve repair may be considered. The current American College of Cardiology (ACC)/American Heart Association valvular heart disease guidelines provide a class IIa recommendation for mitral valve surgery in this setting.[2]

Transcatheter approaches to mitral valve repair have emerged over the past decade as an attractive option in patients who are not candidates for surgical mitral valve repair. Several transcatheter devices for mitral valve repair

No disclosures.

Cleveland Clinic Heart and Vascular Institute, Desk J2-3, 9500 Euclid Avenue, Cleveland, OH 44195, USA

* Corresponding author.

E-mail address: kapadis@ccf.org

Table 1
Common causes of degenerative and functional mitral regurgitation

Degenerative Mitral Regurgitation	Functional Mitral Regurgitation
Prolapse with or without flail	Ischemic cardiomyopathy
Barlow's disease	Dilated cardiomyopathy
Papillary muscle rupture	Hypertrophic cardiomyopathy with systolic anterior motion of the mitral valve
Rheumatic heart disease	
Endocarditis	
Congenital cleft mitral valve	Left atrial enlargement (atrial fibrillation)
Carcinoid heart disease	
Radiation heart disease	

have been developed, including a variety of annuloplasty devices that have gained the Conformité Européenne mark in Europe for use in clinical practice.[3] However, the transcatheter edge-to-edge mitral valve repair device, Mitra-Clip, is the predominant transcatheter mitral valve repair device used in contemporary practice (Fig. 2).

SURGICAL EDGE-TO-EDGE MITRAL VALVE REPAIR

The transcatheter edge-to-edge mitral valve repair device is based on the technique of surgical edge-to-edge repair, in which the anterior and posterior mitral valve leaflets are sutured together at the site of the regurgitant lesion within the coaptation line of the valve.[4] The surgical edge-to-edge repair, or Alfieri stitch, has been well described since the early 1990s. As described by Alfieri and De Bonis, "the key point is to identify the location of the regurgitant jet. Exactly at that point, the free edge of one leaflet is sutured to the corresponding edge of the opposing leaflet thereby eliminating the incompetence of the mitral valve."[4] In patients with a central jet of MR the edge-to-edge repair thus results in a double orifice mitral valve. It is important to carefully assess for intraoperative postrepair mitral valve gradients to be avoid the development of mitral stenosis postrepair.

The surgical edge-to-edge repair technique has been successfully applied broadly to DMR and FMR patients, but mixed results have been reported with surgical edge-to-edge repair for ischemic FMR.[5,6] In a series of 224 patients treated with edge-to-edge repair at a single institution from 1997 to 2001, Bhudia and

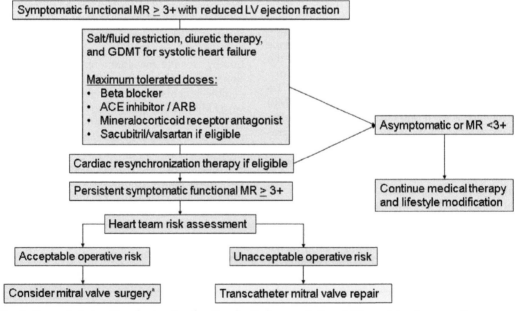

Fig. 1. Suggested algorithm for treating functional mitral regurgitation. ACE, angiotensin converting enzyme; ARB, angiotensin receptor blocker; GDMT, guideline-directed medical therapy; LV, left ventricular; MR, mitral regurgitation. [a] The benefit of mitral valve surgery for the treatment of severe functional mitral regurgitation is uncertain. In addition, the role of transcatheter mitral valve repair or replacement versus mitral valve surgery in patients severe functional mitral regurgitation with acceptable operative risk warrants further investigation.

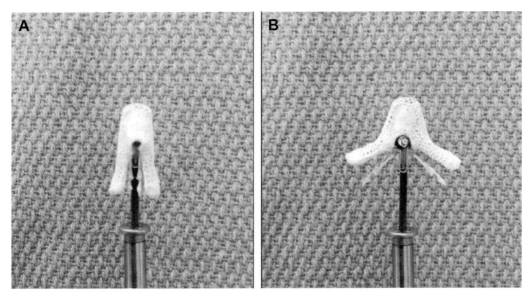

Fig. 2. The MitraClip device. Images of the (A) closed and (B) open MitraClip device. The MitraClip is a cobalt-chromium 2 armed clip covered with a polyester fabric covering.

colleagues[7] observed that edge-to-edge repair offered a significantly less durable repair in patients with ischemic FMR compared with those with either dilated cardiomyopathy or pure DMR. In that series, the proportion of patients with ≥3+ recurrent MR was greater than 20% by 6 months in the ischemic FMR group versus less than 5% in the dilated cardiomyopathy and DMR groups. However, De Bonis and colleagues[6] reported that freedom from repair failure at 1.5 years was 95% among 54 patients with FMR (ischemic and nonischemic) treated with surgical edge-to-edge repair. Encouragingly, a small echocardiographic study of 17 FMR patients with thorough echocardiographic evaluation preoperatively and postoperatively demonstrated that edge-to-edge repair in severe FMR resulted in a major reduction in mitral valve area (8.5 ± 1.9 cm^2 to 3.8 ± 0.9 cm^2, $P<.0001$) with reduced left ventricular size (left ventricular end-diastolic diameter 72 ± 11 mm to 64 ± 10 mm, $P<.01$) and improved left ventricular ejection fraction ($25\% \pm 12\%$ to $38\% \pm 17\%$, $P<.02$).[8] These findings highlight that treatment of severe FMR with an edge-to-edge repair device offers the potential to promote positive remodeling and improved left ventricular performance. This is a central tenet of subsequent trials of transcatheter edge-to-edge mitral valve repair in FMR, in which the device has been tested as a strategy to alleviate adverse consequences of systolic heart failure.

THE MitraClip DEVICE AND PROCEDURE

The MitraClip device (Abbott Medical, Santa Clara, CA) is the predominant transcatheter edge-to-edge mitral valve repair device in use in contemporary practice. The device has been commercially available in Europe since 2008, and was approved by the Food and Drug Administration (FDA) for use in DMR in the United States in 2013. Although many other transcatheter structural interventional procedures (such as transcatheter aortic valve replacement) have moved toward minimalist approaches with conscious sedation, the MitraClip procedure requires general anesthesia and transesophageal echocardiographic guidance given the complexity of the mitral anatomy and the need for outstanding image quality to guide device placement.

The device itself is a cobalt-chromium 2-armed clip covered with polyester fabric (see Fig. 2). The clip is available in 2 sizes, NTR and XTR. The NTR device has a closed clip length of 15 mm, grasping width of 17 mm, and arm length of 9 mm. The larger XTR device offers a closed clip length of 18 mm, grasping width of 22 mm, and arm length of 12 mm. The MitraClip procedure is performed using a transfemoral, transseptal approach. Once femoral venous access is established, the ideal location for puncture of the interatrial septum should be guided by real-time transesophageal echocardiography. A transseptal puncture that is too inferior or too anterior will impede the operator's ability to deliver the device to the valve. Ideally the transseptal puncture should be posterior and superior in the septum to allow at least 4.5 to 5.0 cm of height to deliver the MitraClip device adequately. A standard transseptal catheter and needle can be used to puncture and subsequently deliver a guidewire into the left atrium or left upper pulmonary vein. The patient should be anticoagulated to achieve an activated clotting time of 250 to 300 seconds. The septum is then dilated over a stiff guidewire to allow the 24Fr steerable guide catheter to pass. The clip delivery system is advanced through the steerable guide catheter, and the clip is positioned superior to the site of the most severe MR jet with echocardiographic guidance. The clip is then advanced inferiorly beneath the valve plane, and pulled back with the arms extended to capture the anterior and posterior mitral valve leaflets at the site of the MR jet (Fig. 3). The degree of MR and the measurement of transmitral gradients are then assessed while the clip is in place but before release of the device from the delivery system. If the result is acceptable, the clip is released from the guide catheter. If the result is not optimal, the clip may be reopened and repositioned. After successful repair with the MitraClip device, the mitral valve often has a double orifice anatomy depending on the site of repair (Fig. 4). It is fairly common for multiple clips to be

necessary to achieve a satisfactory result. More than 1 clip was implanted in 34.5% of the 2952 patients treated with commercial MitraClip devices in the United States from 2013 to 2015 in the Society for Thoracic Surgeons (STS)/ACC Transcatheter Valve Therapy registry.[9]

SAFETY AND EFFICACY OF THE MitraClip

The safety and feasibility of the MitraClip was established in the EVEREST (Endovascular Valve Edge-to-edge Repair Study) I clinical trial. In that series of 27 patients treated with the MitraClip for severe MR, the rate of 30-day major adverse events was 15% (1 stroke, 3 clip detachments), but there were 0 deaths at 30 days and all patients were discharged to home. However, in that series only 2/27 (7%) patients had FMR, whereas all others were treated for DMR because of prolapse/flail leaflets.[10]

The subsequent EVEREST II trial was a larger randomized comparison of surgical mitral valve repair or replacement compared with the Mitra-Clip in 279 patients with severe MR.[11] In that study, the primary endpoint of freedom from death, mitral valve surgery, and grade ≥3+ MR at 12 months was significantly higher with surgery (73% vs 55%, P=.007), driven primarily by the need for subsequent mitral valve surgery. However, major adverse events at 30 days

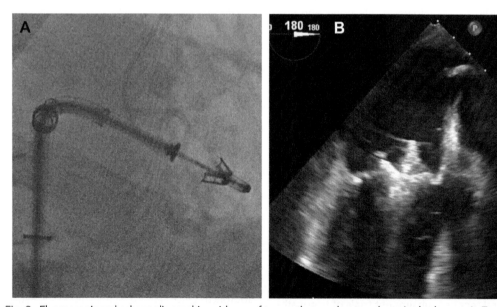

Fig. 3. Fluoroscopic and echocardiographic guidance of transcatheter edge-to-edge mitral valve repair. Transcatheter edge-to-edge mitral valve repair with the MitraClip device requires: (A) fluoroscopic and (B) transesophageal echocardiographic guidance. (A) A right anterior oblique projection of the MitraClip delivery system and device crossing the interatrial septum. The clip arms are extended to capture the anterior and posterior mitral valve leaflets. (B) A 180° transesophageal echocardiographic image of the clip capturing the anterior and posterior mitral valve leaflets before deployment.

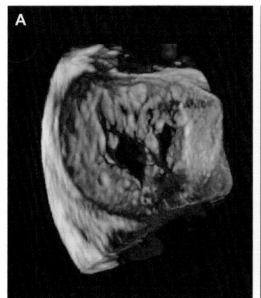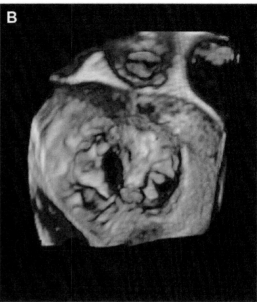

Fig. 4. Double orifice mitral valve after transcatheter edge-to-edge repair. 3D transesophageal echocardiography (A) before and (B) after transcatheter edge-to-edge mitral valve repair with the MitraClip device. (B) A double orifice mitral valve that is expected after edge-to-edge repair of the medial scallop of the anterior and posterior mitral valve leaflets.

were far more common in patients randomized to surgery (48% vs 15%, P<.001), driven primarily by increased need for periprocedural blood transfusion. The finding of lower adverse events in the MitraClip arm in EVEREST II underscores the potential advantages of a transcatheter approach to mitral valve replacement. Approximately 80% of patients treated with MitraClip had moderate or less MR at 12 months follow-up, demonstrating that the device offers at least intermediate-term durability with a significant reduction in the degree of regurgitation, although it does not completely eliminate MR. Patients in both groups had significant reductions in left ventricular dimensions (end-diastolic volume: −25.3 ± 28.3 mL with MitraClip and −40.2 ± 35.9 mL with surgery) and improvements in quality of life at 12 months, further confirming the clinical benefits of the MitraClip. According to subgroup analysis of EVEREST II with regard to the mechanism of MR, patients with FMR demonstrated no significant difference in the primary endpoint between surgery and MitraClip, although surgery was associated with better outcomes in DMR patients. However, 73% of the patients in the trial had DMR, whereas only 27% had FMR.

Whereas the EVEREST II trial enrolled patients who were acceptable operative candidates, the EVEREST II High Risk Study included 78 patients at high risk for open mitral valve surgery who were compared with a retrospective control population of screened patients who were not treated with the device.[12] Although only 27% of the patients enrolled in the EVEREST II study had FMR, 59% of the patients in the High Risk Study had FMR. In that study, procedural success was 96% and 30-day mortality was 7.7%, compared with an estimated 30-day surgical operative mortality of 14.2%. Treatment with the MitraClip was associated with reduced left ventricular size, improved functional capacity and quality of life, and improved survival (1-year survival 76% with MitraClip vs 55% without, P=.047). Longer-term follow-up of the EVEREST II High Risk Study demonstrated that, at 5 years, 75% of patients had MR severity ≤2+ with significant and durable reductions in left ventricular size.[13] The results of the EVEREST II High Risk Study support the safety and efficacy of MitraClip among patients with predominantly FMR who are at high surgical risk.

However, in 2013 the FDA approved the MitraClip for use only in patients with severe symptomatic DMR who are not surgical candidates. This decision was based in part on combined data from 127 patients with severe symptomatic DMR with prohibitive surgical risk treated with MitraClip in the EVEREST II and RE-ALISM (Real World Expanded Multicenter Study of the MitraClip System) High Risk Registry. In that pooled analysis, device success was high (95.3%) and procedural mortality (6.3%) was lower than predicted by the STS risk score for 30-day mortality with mitral valve surgery.[14] Moreover, that analysis revealed improved quality of life and reduced heart failure hospitalizations in patients whose MR severity was reduced. Given the lack of medical therapy options in DMR patients without underlying cardiomyopathy, MitraClip was approved by the FDA in DMR to fulfill an unmet need in this population of inoperable surgical risk patients. However, the initial FDA indication for MitraClip did not include use in FMR owing to the paucity of definitive safety and efficacy data in FMR patients at that time and the potential benefit of medical therapy in FMR patients.[15]

REAL-WORLD EVIDENCE FOR MitraClip IN FUNCTIONAL MITRAL REGURGITATION

In 2013, the same year that the FDA approved the MitraClip in DMR, the early and 1-year results of MitraClip in FMR from the ACCESS-EU registry were reported.[16] This was a prospective evaluation of 567 patients treated with the MitraClip at 14 centers across Europe following commercial approval of the device in 2008. Most patients (69%) were treated for FMR. Although the FMR patients in this study comprised a high-risk group (41% over age 75 years, 71% with congestive heart failure, 33% with prior coronary artery bypass graft surgery, 20% with defibrillators, 66% with left ventricular ejection fraction $\leq$40%, and 48% with logistic euroSCORE $\geq$20%), 30-day procedural complications in FMR patients were very low (mortality 2.8%, stroke 0.5%, major bleeding 3.8%). The ACCESS-EU registry experience also demonstrated major improvements in MR reduction (79% of FMR patients were free of FMR>2+ at 1 year), New York Heart Association functional status, 6-minute walk test, and quality of life as ascertained by the Minnesota Living with Heart Failure Questionnaire. These data further supported the concept that MitraClip may offer an alternative to mitral valve surgery in high- or prohibitive-risk patients with severe FMR.

Further data regarding commercial MitraClip use in the United States followed in 2017 with results from the STS/ACC Transcatheter Valve Therapy Registry. The MitraClip was used in 2952 patients across 145 US Centers during the first 2 years of commercial FDA approval, and 1867 patients with linked Centers for Medicare and Medicaid Services claims data were analyzed.[9] Only a minority of patients were treated with pure FMR (8.6%) or mixed DMR/FMR (8.9%). This is likely a consequence of the more narrow DMR approval for the device in the United States compared with the European experience. This 1-year cumulative incidence of mortality (24.7% vs 31.2%, P=.02), heart failure hospitalization (20.5% vs 32.6%, P=.008), and mortality or heart failure hospitalization (35.7% vs 49.0%, P=.002) were significantly lower in DMR patients versus FMR patients. However, the differences in these endpoints may be confounded by important differences in the baseline risk of the DMR and FMR populations enrolled in the registry. This was confirmed by the observation that, on multivariate analysis, FMR was not significantly associated with 1-year mortality or the composite of 1-year mortality or heart failure hospitalization. Increasing age, dialysis, moderate or severe lung disease, severe tricuspid regurgitation, and postprocedure MR > grade 2+ were independently associated with 1 year mortality.

RANDOMIZED CLINICAL TRIALS OF MitraClip IN FUNCTIONAL MITRAL REGURGITATION

Although observational evidence supported the use of MitraClip in FMR, randomized clinical trial evidence was necessary to confirm these findings and to support commercial FDA approval in the United States. In 2018, 2 pivotal trials—MITRA-FR (Multicentre Randomized Study of Percutaneous Mitral Valve Repair MitraClip Device in Patients With Severe Secondary Mitral Regurgitation) and COAPT (Clinical Outcomes Assessment of the MitraClip Percutaneous Therapy for High Surgical Risk Patients)—were published and will shape the future use of the MitraClip device in clinical practice and its prospects for FDA approval in FMR patients (Table 2).

MITRA-FR

The MITRA-FR trial randomized 307 patients with severe, symptomatic FMR and reduced ejection fraction (15%–40%) to MitraClip with medical therapy or medical therapy alone.[17] Only patients deemed inoperable for mitral valve surgery were eligible. This was an open label trial that was conducted at 37 centers in France. Each center was required to have performed at least 5 MitraClip procedures before inclusion in the study. Patients included in the trial were typical for a high-risk surgical

Table 2
Comparison of the MITRA-FR and COAPT trials

	MITRA-FR[17]	COAPT[18]
Population	Severe FMR with LVEF 15%–40% deemed inoperable by heart team	≥Moderately severe FMR with LVEF 20%–50% deemed inoperable by heart team
Sites	37 centers in France	78 centers in North America
N	307	614
Severe MR criteria	EROA >20 mm^2 or RV >30 mL	Grade ≥3 + by echo core lab
Methodology	1:1 randomized trial of medical therapy with or without MitraClip	1:1 randomized trial of maximum tolerated medical therapy with or without MitraClip
Primary efficacy endpoint	All-cause death or unplanned HF hospitalization within 12 mo: 54.6% with vs 51.3% without MitraClip ($P = .53$)	All hospitalization for HF within 24 mo: annualized rate of 35.8% with vs 67.9% without MitraClip ($P<.001$)
1-y all-cause death	24.3% with vs 22.4% without MitraClip	19.1% with vs 23.2% without MitraClip ($P<.001$)
Key secondary endpoints	• 1 y CV death: 21.7% with vs 20.4% without MitraClip • 1 y unplanned HF hospitalization: 48.7% with vs 47.4% without MitraClip • 1 y MACE: 56.6% with vs 51.3% without MitraClip	• 1 y MR grade ≤2+: 94.8% with vs 46.9% without MitraClip, $P<.001$ • 1 y change in 6MWT (min): −2.2 ± 9.1 with vs −60.2 ± 9.0 without MitraClip, $P<.001$ • 1 y NYHA class ≤2: 72.2% with vs 49.6% without MitraClip, $P<.001$ • 1 y change in LVEDV (mL): −3.7 ± 5.1 with vs +17.1 ± 5.1 without MitraClip, $P = .004$
Key safety endpoints in MitraClip arm	• Device failure: 4.2% • Transfusion-dependent bleeding or vascular injury requiring surgery: 3.5% • Atrial septum lesion or defect: 2.8% • Cardiac embolism and/or stroke: 1.4% • Tamponade: 1.4% • Urgent surgery: 0%	• 30-d freedom from death, stroke, MI, and nonelective CV surgery for device complications: 96.9% • Primary safety endpoint – 1 y freedom from device-related complications: 94.8%

Abbreviations: 6MWT, 6-min walk test; CV, cardiovascular; EROA, effective regurgitant orifice area; FMR, functional mitral regurgitation; HF, heart failure; LVEDV, left ventricular end-diastolic volume; LVEF, left ventricular ejection fraction; MACE, major adverse cardiac events; MI, myocardial infarction; MR, mitral regurgitation; NYHA, New York Heart Association; RV, right ventricle.

population with a mean age of 70 years, 59% with ischemic cardiomyopathy, mean left ventricular ejection fraction of 33%, and reduced renal function (mean glomerular filtration rate of 48–50 mL/min). The primary outcome, a composite of death or unplanned heart failure hospitalization at 12 months, was similar in both groups (54.6% with MitraClip vs 51.3% without MitraClip; $P=.53$). Secondary outcomes (all-cause death, cardiovascular death, unplanned heart failure hospitalization, major adverse cardiovascular events) were also similar between groups. These results, published in August of 2018, called into question the effectiveness of percutaneous mitral valve repair as a treatment of severe symptomatic FMR among inoperable patients.

COAPT

However, the following month the results of the COAPT (Cardiovascular Outcomes Assessment of the MitraClip Percutaneous Therapy for Heart Failure Patients With Functional Mitral Regurgitation) Trial were presented at the 2018 Transcatheter Cardiovascular Therapeutic scientific meeting. The COAPT trial was also an open label, randomized controlled trial in which 614 patients with moderate-to-severe symptomatic FMR with reduced left ventricular ejection fraction (20%–50%) were randomized to MitraClip with guideline-directed medical therapy or to guideline-directed medical therapy alone.[18] Similar to the MITRA-FR study, only patients who were deemed not candidates for mitral valve surgery were eligible for inclusion. The patient population also had a mean age of 72.5 years, 61% with ischemic cardiomyopathy, mean left ventricular ejection fraction of 31%, and 73% with creatinine clearance $\leq$60 mL/min. The primary outcome, all hospitalization for heart failure within 24 months, was significantly reduced in the MitraClip arm (35.8% vs 67.9%, $P<.001$), as were each of the hierarchical secondary endpoints that included metrics of MR severity, quality of life, functional status, left ventricular size, and all-cause death at 2 years, which was 29.1% in the MitraClip arm versus 46.1% in the control arm ($P<.001$). The findings of COAPT were overwhelmingly positive in favor of the MitraClip device as an important tool in the treatment of severe FMR among inoperable patients.

Contrasting MITRA-FR and COAPT

The MITRA-FR and COAPT trials provide conflicting results on the role of MitraClip in FMR patients. Although similar in design, these trials have important differences that may have contributed to the varying results. First, there were differences in the severity of MR in the enrolled patient populations. The mean effective regurgitant orifice area was 31 mL in MITRA-FR compared with 41 mL in COAPT; furthermore, left ventricular volumes were significantly larger among the patients in MITRA-FR compared with COAPT. Therefore, the patient population in MITRA-FR had less severe MR and larger ventricles, which may reflect a population in which MR is not a major driver of poor outcomes. Second, there were differences in the success of the MitraClip procedures in the trials. In MITRA-FR, 9% of the device arm did not receive a MitraClip device because of procedural failure or other reasons compared 5% of patients in the device arm of COAPT. Third, among the patients who did receive a MitraClip, the acute results seem to be slightly better in the COAPT trial. In MITRA-FR, 8.1% of the device arm patients had MR $\geq$3+ after MitraClip, whereas that rate was 4% in COAPT. The MitraClip device seemed to have a more favorable safety profile in the COAPT trial: the rate of periprocedural complications was 14.6% in the MITRA-FR trial, whereas the rate of device-related complications

at 12 months was only 3.4% in the COAPT trial. The signal of improved device success and safety in COAPT may relate to the improved effectiveness of the therapy observed in that trial compared with the less favorable MITRA-FR results. Finally, patients in the COAPT trial were symptomatic, with severe MR despite maximally tolerated, guideline-directed medical therapy (including cardiac resynchronization therapy, as indicated) under the direction of a heart failure specialist; the medical therapy in both arms did not change substantially over the course of the trial. This suggests that the COAPT trial may have selected the FMR patient population who would benefit most from transcatheter mitral valve repair.

In March 2019, the MitraClip gained FDA approval for commercial use in the US among patients with severe FMR, providing a highly anticipated new tool in the toolbox of treatments for FMR.

SUMMARY AND FUTURE DIRECTIONS

Transcatheter valvular heart interventions have rapidly expanded over the past 2 decades. These developments have led to promising new devices that offer the potential to improve symptoms, quality of life, and survival in patients with severe FMR who are not candidates for cardiac surgery. The MitraClip device is the predominant transcatheter mitral device in contemporary practice, with a growing body of real-world and clinical trial evidence to support its use in DMR and FMR. However, there remain certain anatomic issues that may preclude technically successful transcatheter edge-to-edge mitral valve repair, including: (1) severe mitral annular calcification compromising mitral valve area, (2) severely restricted mitral valve leaflets, (3) severe leaflet calcification, (4) cleft leaflets, and (5) very small posterior mitral valve leaflet. In addition, loss of leaflet insertion in the MitraClip device contributes to recurrence of clinically important MR, and these patients have low rates of success of repeat MitraClip procedures (25% procedural success in 1 series).[19] Several novel transcatheter mitral valve repair devices are currently in various stages of development. Future work is needed to understand the safety, effectiveness, and durability of these devices and their application in populations not amenable to edge-to-edge repair devices. In addition, as transcatheter mitral valve interventions continue to mature, it remains to be seen which patients will be best suited by transcatheter mitral valve repair versus replacement.

REFERENCES

1. Nkomo VT, Gardin JM, Skelton TN, et al. Burden of valvular heart diseases: a population-based study. Lancet 2006;368:1005–11.

2. Nishimura RA, Otto CM, Bonow RO, et al. 2014 AHA/ACC guideline for the management of patients with valvular heart disease: executive summary: a report of the American College of Cardiology/American Heart Association Task Force on practice guidelines. J Am Coll Cardiol 2014;63:2438–88.

3. Figulla HR, Webb JG, Lauten A, et al. The transcatheter valve technology pipeline for treatment of adult valvular heart disease. Eur Heart J 2016; 37:2226–39.

4. Alfieri O, De Bonis M. The role of the edge-to-edge repair in the surgical treatment of mitral regurgitation. J Card Surg 2010;25:536–41.

5. Maisano F, Torracca L, Oppizzi M, et al. The edge-to-edge technique: a simplified method to correct mitral insufficiency. Eur J Cardiothorac Surg 1998; 13:240–5 [discussion: 245–6].

6. De Bonis M, Lapenna E, La Canna G, et al. Mitral valve repair for functional mitral regurgitation in end-stage dilated cardiomyopathy: role of the "edge-to-edge" technique. Circulation 2005;112:I402–8.

7. Bhudia SK, McCarthy PM, Smedira NG, et al. Edge-to-edge (Alfieri) mitral repair: results in diverse clinical settings. Ann Thorac Surg 2004;77:1598–606.

8. Kinnaird TD, Munt BI, Ignaszewski AP, et al. Edge-to-edge repair for functional mitral regurgitation: an echocardiographic study of the hemodynamic consequences. J Heart Valve Dis 2003;12:280–6.

9. Sorajja P, Vemulapalli S, Feldman T, et al. Outcomes with transcatheter mitral valve repair in the united states: an STS/ACC TVT registry report. J Am Coll Cardiol 2017;70:2315–27.

10. Feldman T, Wasserman HS, Herrmann HC, et al. Percutaneous mitral valve repair using the edge-to-edge technique: six-month results of the EVEREST phase I clinical trial. J Am Coll Cardiol 2005;46:2134–40.

11. Feldman T, Foster E, Glower DD, et al. Percutaneous repair or surgery for mitral regurgitation. N Engl J Med 2011;364:1395–406.

12. Whitlow PL, Feldman T, Pedersen WR, et al. Acute and 12-month results with catheter-based mitral valve leaflet repair: the EVEREST II (Endovascular Valve Edge-to-Edge Repair) high risk study. J Am Coll Cardiol 2012;59:130–9.

13. Kar S, Feldman T, Qasim A, et al. Five-year outcomes of transcatheter reduction of significant mitral regurgitation in high-surgical-risk patients. Heart 2018. https://doi.org/10.1136/heartjnl-2017-312605.

14. Lim DS, Reynolds MR, Feldman T, et al. Improved functional status and quality of life in prohibitive surgical risk patients with degenerative mitral regurgitation after transcatheter mitral valve repair. J Am Coll Cardiol 2014;64:182–92.

15. MitraClip instructions for use. 2013:1–54.

16. Maisano F, Franzen O, Baldus S, et al. Percutaneous mitral valve interventions in the real world: early and 1-year results from the ACCESS-EU, a prospective, multicenter, nonrandomized postapproval study of the MitraClip therapy in Europe. J Am Coll Cardiol 2013;62:1052–61.

17. Obadia JF, Messika-Zeitoun D, Leurent G, et al. Percutaneous repair or medical treatment for secondary mitral regurgitation. N Engl J Med 2018; 379(24):2297–306.

18. Stone GW, Lindenfeld J, Abraham WT, et al. Transcatheter mitral-valve repair in patients with heart failure. N Engl J Med 2018;379(24): 2307–18.

19. Kreidel F, Frerker C, Schluter M, et al. Repeat MitraClip therapy for significant recurrent mitral regurgitation in high surgical risk patients: impact of loss of leaflet insertion. JACC Cardiovasc Interv 2015;8: 1480–9.

Transcatheter Edge-to-Edge Repair for Primary (Degenerative) Mitral Regurgitation: Registries and Trials

Dhaval Desai, MD, Matthew J. Price, MD*

KEYWORDS

• MitraClip • Mitral regurgitation • Mitral repair • Transcatheter edge-to-edge repair

---

KEY POINTS

- At present, the MitraClip is the only approved transcatheter edge-to-edge repair device that is commercially available for the treatment of severe, symptomatic, primary (degenerative) mitral regurgitation in patients deemed to be at prohibitive risk by a heart team.
- Prospective, observational registries and randomized trials show that transcatheter edge-to-edge repair can be safely performed with a low rate of periprocedural adverse events despite a predominantly elderly patient population with multiple comorbidities.
- Transcatheter edge-to-edge repair is associated with improvement in mitral regurgitation severity, left ventricular dimensions and remodeling, heart failure rehospitalizations, and, in high-risk groups, an improvement in survival compared with medical therapy.
- Risk factors for death or heart failure rehospitalization after transcatheter edge-to-edge repair for primary mitral regurgitation include 3+ or 4+ residual mitral regurgitation, older age, severe tricuspid regurgitation, moderate to severe lung disease, and the need for dialysis.

INTRODUCTION

The mechanism of mitral regurgitation (MR) can be broadly classified into 2 categories: primary (degenerative MR [DMR]) and secondary (functional). In primary MR, the cause of regurgitation is involvement of the mitral leaflets or apparatus, commonly caused by fibroelastic deficiency, whereas, in secondary MR, the leaflets and apparatus are not abnormal but regurgitation occurs because of left ventricular (LV) remodeling, which leads to poor coaptation. The approach and response to treatment may differ substantially between the two entities. Transcatheter edge-to-edge repair with the MitraClip device (Abbott Vascular, Santa Clara, CA) can be used to address primary MR. The device was approved in Europe in March 2008 and became commercially available in September 2008. This device was approved in the United States in October 2013 for the sole application of the treatment of severe, symptomatic, DMR in those patients deemed to be at prohibitive surgical risk by a heart team.[1] This article reviews the registries and trials that explore the short-term and long-term safety and efficacy of transcatheter edge-to-edge repair with the MitraClip in the setting of DMR.

STUDIES PERFORMED WITHIN THE UNITED STATES

Endovascular Valve Edge-to-edge Repair Study Phase I Clinical Trial

The EVEREST (Endovascular Valve Edge-to-edge Repair Study) phase I clinical trial was the first US clinical experience with percutaneous edge-to-edge mitral valve repair.[2] The study enrolled

---

Division of Cardiovascular Diseases, Scripps Clinic, 9898 Genesee Avenue, AMP-200, La Jolla, CA 92037, USA
* Corresponding author.
E-mail address: price.matthew@scrippshealth.org

Intervent Cardiol Clin 8 (2019) 245–259
https://doi.org/10.1016/j.iccl.2019.02.007

55 patients with moderate to severe (3+) or severe (4+) MR. The patients underwent percutaneous repair with the MitraClip system (Abbott, Menlo Park, CA). Key exclusion criteria included LV ejection fraction (LVEF) less than 30%, LV end-systolic dimension (LVESD) more than 55 mm, mitral leaflet coaptation length of less than 2 mm, mitral leaflet coaptation depth more than 11 mm, or recent myocardial infarction within 14 days. All patients were candidates for open mitral valve surgery. The primary end point was defined as a composite of freedom from death, myocardial infarction, cardiac tamponade, need for cardiac surgery, clip detachment, stroke, or sepsis. The efficacy goal was defined as MR severity of less than or equal to 2+ after clip placement.

The first report from this study presented data from 27 of the first 55 patients. The average patient age was 69 years and 59% were male. Device implantation was successful in 24 out of 27 patients; 1 clip was implanted in 20 patients and 2 clips in 4 patients. The primary end point was achieved in 23 of the 27 patients (85%); in 3 patients, a clip could not be implanted and 1 patient had a nonembolic stroke. An additional 3 patients required surgical mitral valve repair. There were no instances of clip embolization. MR less than or equal to 2+ was achieved in 64% patients at 1 month and 59% at 6 months.

Several take-home points were made from this phase I study. The device clearly had a steep learning curve as shown by significant anesthesia, fluoroscopy, and echocardiography times. Also certain cases may require implantation of more than 1 clip to achieve a satisfactory reduction in MR. The degree of residual MR was maintained over the follow-up period for those individuals who had MR less than or equal to 2+ at 1 month.

A subsequent report included 107 patients comprising the 55 patients treated in the EVEREST phase I feasibility trial and the 52 roll-in patients treated in the EVEREST II trial, a randomized controlled trial.[3] These patients were followed for as long as 3 years. The median age was 71 years and 62% of the patients were male; 61% received 1 clip, 29% received 2 clips, and 10% received no clips. Procedure duration decreased over time. Patients remained hemodynamically stable during the procedure; hypotension or ventricular arrhythmias were rarely observed. Major adverse events occurred in 9% of patients (10 patients); these included bleeding requiring more than 2 units of blood transfusion (4 patients), transseptal complications (3 patients), mechanical ventilation for more than 48 hours (2 patients), and death unrelated to device (1 patient). A total 93% of patients were discharged home. The average length of hospital stay was 3.2 days. Partial clip detachment (single leaflet device attachment [SLDA]) occurred in 10 patients at various times over follow-up: 3 during the procedure, 1 before hospital discharge, 5 between discharge and first 30 days, and 1 after 30 days. Acute procedural success, defined as MR severity less than or equal to 2+, was achieved in 74% of patients. At 12 months, 66% of patients showed MR less than or equal to 2+, and 70% remained free from mitral valve surgery over the follow-up.

Technical inexperience may have contributed to the rates of early and late failure, because 70% of the procedures performed represented the first 3 procedures of the participating centers. These initial feasibility studies paved way for the landmark, randomized control trial of edge-to-edge repair for mitral valve regurgitation (EVEREST II).

Endovascular Valve Edge-to-edge Repair Study II Trial

EVEREST II was the landmark trial that in part led to the commercial approval of the MitraClip device in the United States. The trial randomly assigned 279 patients with 3+ or 4+ MR in a 2:1 ratio to treatment with either transcatheter mitral valve repair with the MitraClip or open mitral valve surgery (either repair or replacement) across 37 centers in the United States and Canada.[4] The study only included those patients with malcoaptation of the middle scallop of the anterior and posterior leaflets (ie, A2 and P2). The primary end point was a composite of freedom from death, surgery for mitral valve dysfunction, and 3+ or 4+ MR at 12 months. Secondary end points included change in LV dimensions and volumes, New York Heart Failure Association (NYHA) functional class, and quality-of-life measures. The trial also assessed safety end points at 30 days, which included death, myocardial infarction, reoperation from failed mitral valve surgery, nonelective cardiovascular surgery for adverse events, renal failure, stroke, deep wound infection, mechanical ventilation for more than 48 hours, gastrointestinal complication requiring surgery, new-onset atrial fibrillation, septicemia, and transfusion of 2 or more units.

Asymptomatic patients were eligible for enrollment if they had an ejection fraction between 25% and 60%, LVESD of 40 to 55 mm, new-onset atrial fibrillation, or new-onset pulmonary hypertension. Symptomatic patients were required to have an ejection fraction greater than or equal to 25% and an LVESD less than or equal to 55 mm.

A total of 184 patients were assigned to the percutaneous repair and 95 were assigned to the surgical repair; 21 patients withdrew consent, resulting in 258 remaining patients, of whom 243 patients (94%) complied with the protocol and achieved 12-month follow-up. The average patient age was 67.3 years in the percutaneous repair group and 65.7 years in the surgery group; about 30% of the patients in both groups were aged 75 years or older. Most of the patients had NYHA II or III heart failure. Patients with both DMR (primary) and functional (secondary) MR were enrolled, and the cause of MR was degenerative in approximately three-quarters of the study population. In the surgery group, 86% of patients were treated with mitral valve repair and 14% of patients had mitral valve replacement. In the transcatheter repair arm, according to intention to treat, freedom from death, surgery for mitral valve dysfunction, and grade 3+ or 4+ MR at 12 months was achieved in 55% of patients undergoing percutaneous repair and 73% in surgical repair group ($P = .007$). In a per-protocol analysis, the primary end point was achieved in 72% of patients undergoing percutaneous repair versus 88% in the surgery group ($P = .02$). This difference was driven entirely by the need for surgery for mitral valve dysfunction (20% in percutaneous repair vs 2% in surgical repair). The death rate at 12 months was 6% for both groups and residual 3+ or 4+ MR at 12 months was also similar (21% vs 20%). Major adverse events within the first 30 days occurred more frequently in the surgery group, driven by the need for blood transfusions (13% vs 45%). Secondary analyses showed that percutaneous repair resulted in greater preservation of LV function and lesser decrease in LV dimensions compared with surgery. Quality of life and NYHA class were better after the percutaneous repair compared with surgery.

The EVEREST II population was followed for 5 years and interim 4-year and 5-year results were published in 2013 and 2015, respectively.[5,6] A total of 87% of patients in the percutaneous arm and 70% of patients in the surgical arm were included in the 5-year analysis. Failure to implant the device occurred in 9.5% of the patients and SLDA occurred in 6.3% of the procedures. The primary end point still favored the surgical arm: freedom from death, surgery for mitral valve dysfunction, and 3+ or 4+ residual MR at 5 years occurred in 64.3% in the surgical arm and 44.2% in the percutaneous repair arm. There was no difference in the rate of death between surgery and percutaneous repair (20.8% vs 26.8%; $P = .36$); however, the rate of 3+ or 4+ MR was significantly greater with percutaneous repair (12.3% vs 1.8%; $P = .02$), as was the need for surgery or reoperation (27.9% vs 8.9%; $P = .003$). According to landmark analysis, freedom from mitral valve surgery or reoperation remained the same after percutaneous repair or surgery beyond 6 months of the procedure (**Fig. 1**). Improvements in symptoms and LV dimensions were maintained at 5 years in both study arms. The treatment effect of surgery seemed to be heterogeneous, because a significant interaction was observed among

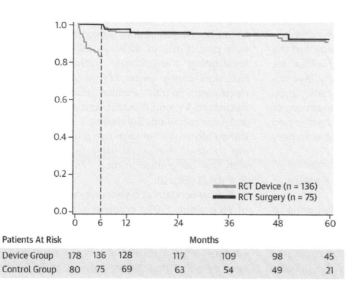

Patients At Risk							
	0	6	12	24	36	48	60
Device Group	178	136	128	117	109	98	45
Control Group	80	75	69	63	54	49	21

Legend: RCT Device (n = 136); RCT Surgery (n = 75)

Fig. 1. Landmark analysis of freedom from mitral valve surgery or reoperation beyond 6 months after transcatheter edge-to-edge repair or open surgery in the EVEREST II randomized clinical trial (RCT). (*From* Feldman T, Kar S, Elmariah S, et al. Randomized comparison of percutaneous repair and surgery for mitral regurgitation 5-year results of EVEREST II. J Am Coll Cardiol 2015;66(25):2844–54; with permission.)

patients greater than 70 years of age, those with functional mechanism for MR, and those with LVEF less than 60%. The benefit of surgery seemed to be greater in younger patients and those with normal ejection fraction, whereas the results seemed comparable between surgery and percutaneous repair in the elderly and those with functional MR.

The EVEREST II study has several limitations. For example, more patients within the surgical arm withdrew from the study before undergoing mitral valve surgery. Most operators had little, if any, experience with the MitraClip procedure, whereas the cardiothoracic surgeons were experienced and from top surgical centers. Most patients in the percutaneous arm received only 1 clip, and the protocol mandated at most 2 clips, which differs from current MitraClip techniques and the current MitraClip experience as seen in the Transcatheter Valve Therapy (TVT) registry. Also, part of the superior improvement in MR in the surgical arm may have been caused by the addition of an annuloplasty ring in addition to mitral valve repair; 38 of the 69 surgical repair patients underwent leaflet restriction and annuloplasty, 16 of 69 patients underwent annuloplasty alone, and 14 of 69 patients underwent complex leaflet or chordal repair with annuloplasty.

In conclusion, the results from EVEREST II show that percutaneous repair is safe in patients with 3+ or 4+ MR and the option for surgical repair still remained viable in these individuals if percutaneous repair failed. Positive effects on LV remodeling and durability of percutaneous repair were seen in long-term follow-up. Also, if patients remained event free within the initial 6 months after percutaneous repair, freedom from mitral valve surgery or reoperation was similar to surgical repair. This study, in combination with the EVEREST II High Risk Study and the REALISM (Real World Expanded Multicenter Study of the MitraClip System) registry, eventually led to the US Food and Drug Administration (FDA) approval of the MitraClip for treatment of significant DMR ($\geq$3+) in those patients deemed to be at prohibitive risk for mitral valve surgery as determined by a heart team.[1]

Endovascular Valve Edge-to-edge Repair Study II High Risk Study

The EVEREST High Risk Study enrolled patients with 3+ or 4+ MR at prohibitive surgical risk, defined as an estimated perioperative mortality of greater than or equal to 12% according to the Society of Thoracic Surgeons (STS) risk score or by the estimation of the surgeon investigator

based on prespecified criteria.[7] These high-risk criteria included mobile atheroma of the ascending aorta, postmediastinal radiation, age older than 75 years with LVEF<40%, hepatic cirrhosis, prior median sternotomy with bypass grafts, or a creatinine level greater than 2.5 mg/dL. Key exclusion criteria included recent myocardial infarction, LVEF less than 20%, LVESD greater than 60 mm, or leaflet anatomy that might affect device implantation. A total of 78 patients were enrolled, and were compared with a 36-patient concurrent comparator group (control) that consisted of patients who fulfilled inclusion criteria but who did not enroll in the study or were not anatomically eligible for device implantation. The average age of the two groups was 77 years. The mean predicted surgical mortality based on calculated STS risk score was 14.2% in the high-risk group and 14.9% in the concurrent comparator group. More than half the patients had prior cardiovascular surgery and about 90% of patients had NYHA class III or IV symptoms. The cause of MR was functional in 59% and degenerative in 41% of patients. The clip was successfully implanted in 96% of the patients (75 out of 78 patients); 1 patient had intracardiac thrombus, 1 had a transseptal complication, and 1 patient's MR was unable to be treated with clip. The rate of major adverse events at 30 days was 27% (21 of 78 patients): 14 needed transfusion of greater than or equal to 2 units of blood, 3 developed renal failure, 2 experienced major stroke, 2 needed more than 48 hours of mechanical ventilation, and 6 died. At least a 1-grade reduction in MR was achieved in 79.5% of cases, and MR grade less than or equal to 2+ was achieved in 71.8%. The rate of heart failure hospitalization was significantly lower in the year following MitraClip implantation compared with the year prior (16% vs 42%; P<.02). The patients undergoing transcatheter mitral valve repair had significantly better NYHA functional class, decreased mitral annular dimensions, and decreased LV end-diastolic and systolic volume at 1-year follow-up. Survival at 1 year was significantly higher in the high-risk patients undergoing transcatheter mitral valve repair compared with the comparator group (76.4% vs 55.3%; P = .047) (Fig. 2).[7]

Follow-up data at 5 years were available in 70 of 78 patients (90%) enrolled in the EVEREST II High Risk Study.[8] Survival at 1, 3, and 5 years was 76%, 59%, and 43%, respectively. Those who had acute procedural success (residual MR severity $\leq$2+) had better survival at 1, 3, and 5 years compared with those who had MR

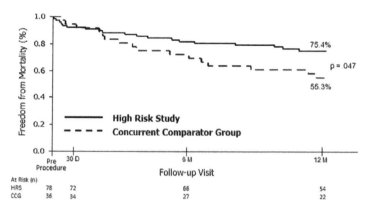

Fig. 2. Kaplan-Meier curve of survival after transcatheter edge-edge-repair compared with medical therapy in patients at very high risk for open mitral valve surgery in the EVEREST II High Risk Study. (*From* Whitlow PL, Feldman T, Pedersen WR, et al. Acute and 12-month results with catheter-based mitral valve leaflet repair: the EVEREST II (Endovascular Valve Edge-to-Edge Repair) high risk study. J Am Coll Cardiol 2012;59(2):130–9; with permission.)

severity greater than or equal to 3+. Survival benefit was inversely proportional to severity of MR at discharge; those with 0+/1+ MR at discharge had better survival compared with more than 2+ MR at discharge. For those patients that were alive at 5 years, 75% had MR less than or equal to 2%. The MitraClip procedure showed sustained MR reduction over follow-up, along with significant and sustained reductions in LV end-diastolic volume (LVEDV) and LV end-systolic volume (LVESV) at 5 years. The reductions in LVEDV and LVESV also correlated in improvement in NYHA class: at 1 year, 74% had NYHA class I or II, whereas at 5 years 83% had NYHA class I or II. Very few patients required surgery (2.6%) or reinterventions (2.6%) over 5-year follow-up.

Endovascular Valve Edge-to-edge Repair Study II Real World Expanded Multicenter Study of the MitraClip System Study

REALISM was a prospective, multicenter, continued access registry designed to continue to collect data to further assess the safety and effectiveness of the MitraClip device after the EVEREST II randomized trial completed enrollment. Included patients were both high risk and non–high risk for open surgery.[9] The primary clinical end point was a composite of death, myocardial infarction, reoperation for failed surgical repair or replacement, nonelective cardiovascular surgery for adverse events, stroke, renal failure, deep wound infection, ventilation for greater than 48 hours, gastrointestinal complication requiring surgery, new onset of permanent atrial fibrillation, septicemia, and transfusion of 2 units of blood or more. The efficacy end point was defined as freedom from surgery for MR or valve dysfunction, death, and MR grade 3+ or 4+ at 12 months.

The non–high-risk arm consisted of 271 patients, 85% of whom were 65 years of age or older, and the mean age was 74 years. The primary end point occurred in 31 patients (11.4%) at 30 days and 74 patients (27.3%) at 12 months. The 12-month efficacy end point in the non–high-risk arm was achieved in 66.9% of patients. The average age of the 628 patients in the high-risk arm was 76.7 years, and 60% were male. The primary end point occurred in 98 patients (15.6%) at 30 days and 223 patients (35.5%) at 12 months. The 12-month efficacy end point was achieved in 61% of patients.

The EVEREST Investigators specifically looked at the 127 patients at prohibitive surgical risk with primary MR (DMR) from the EVEREST II High Risk and REALISM High Risk cohorts,[10] defined as an STS predicted risk of operative mortality (STS-PROM) greater than or equal to 8% for mitral valve replacement or the presence of high-risk characteristics as outlined in the EVEREST II High Risk Study inclusion criteria. Of these 127 patients, 25 patients were from the EVEREST II High Risk Registry and 98 patients were from the high-risk arm of the REALISM continued access registry.

The average age of this study population was 82 years, 83.5% of patients were more than 75 years of age, 55% were male, 73% had a history of coronary artery disease, 71% had atrial fibrillation, and 48% of patients had prior cardiovascular surgery. The included patients were symptomatic as well as at high surgical risk, because 87% of patients were in NYHA class III or IV at time of enrollment and the mean STS score was 13.2%. The MitraClip was successfully implanted in 121 patients (95.3%); acute procedural success, defined as 2+ or less MR, was achieved in 98 patients (78%). The average hospital stay was approximately 3 days and nearly

90% of patients were discharged to home. Of those patients discharged with grade 2+ or less MR, 70.3% had grade 2+ or less MR at 12 months. The 30-day and 12-month mortalities were 6.3% and 23.6% respectively. LV dimensions, NYHA class, heart failure hospitalizations, and quality of life were all improved at 12 months. The favorable results of MitraClip in EVEREST II and EVEREST II High Risk Study led to the FDA approval of the use of this device in symptomatic patients with DMR who are at prohibitive risk for surgical mitral valve intervention.

Transcatheter Valve Therapy Registry

In August of 2014, the Centers for Medicare & Medicaid Services (CMS) issued a National Coverage Determination that allows for coverage of transcatheter mitral valve repair under Coverage with Evidence Development with several conditions, including participation in the prospective, national, audited STS/American College of Cardiology (ACC) TVT registry. The goal of this registry is to measure several parameters that will lead to quality assurance and improvement initiatives, efficient conduction of new studies, and possible expansion of device labeling through evidence development. The results of the initial commercial US experience were made available in 2016.[11] Patients who underwent percutaneous repair from November 2013 to August 2014 were included; patients enrolled in research studies were excluded. Patients had symptomatic, moderate-to-severe or severe primary MR and were deemed to be prohibitive surgical risk by a cardiac surgeon and cardiologist. Prohibitive risk was defined as STS-PROM score of either greater than or equal to 6% risk for mitral valve repair or greater than or equal to 8% risk for isolated mitral valve replacement or the presence of clinical factors not captured in the risk calculator algorithm (similar to the EVEREST II High Risk cohort). Both in-hospital and 30-day outcomes were examined. The primary outcome analyzed was postimplantation MR severity of 2+ or less without conversion to open cardiac surgery and without in-hospital mortality. A total 564 patients from 61 hospitals were evaluated: the median age was 83 years, 56% were male, 86% of patients were NYHA III or IV functional class, 30% had prior PCI, 39% had 1 or more prior cardiac surgeries, and 15% were oxygen dependent. The mean STS-PROM score was 7.9% for mitral valve repair and 10% for mitral valve replacement. The mechanism of MR was degenerative (primary) in 85% and mixed (both primary

and secondary) in 5% of patients (29 of 564). Participating hospitals performed a median number of 6 procedures during the study period. Technical success was frequent, because a MitraClip was implanted in 96.8% of procedures and an MR grade of 2+ or less was achieved in 93% of the patients. Only 3 patients (0.5%) required conversion to open cardiac surgery. In-hospital death occurred in 13 patients (2.3%); 4 of these deaths (0.7%) were cardiac related. Overall in-hospital procedural success (2+ or less MR without need for cardiac surgery or in-hospital mortality) was 91%. Procedural complications occurred in 45 patients (8%); major bleeding accounted for approximately half. Other complications included a 30-day stroke rate of 1.8%, an SLDA rate of 1.1%, and a device embolization rate of 0.4%. Overall in-hospital procedural success (2+ or less MR without need for cardiac surgery or in-hospital mortality) was 91%. Median length of stay was 3 days, 84% were discharged home, and 10% were discharged to extended care.

At 30-days, the rate of all-cause mortality at was 5.8%, and the rate of cardiovascular mortality was 2.6%. Overall 30-day procedural success (2+ or less MR without need for cardiac surgery or 30-day mortality) was 86%. Predictors of MR reduction included smaller LV end-diastolic dimension, lower severity of baseline MR, MR involving the A2-P2 scallops of mitral valve, and higher institutional case volume. Fig. 3 shows the change in MR following transcatheter repair and summarizes the occurrence of major adverse clinical events.[11]

Results from the TVT registry were reported again in 2017.[12] This report encompassed patients undergoing transcatheter mitral valve repair in the United States from November 2013 to September 1, 2015. A total of 2952 patients treated at 145 hospitals were included in the study and 1867 of the patients (63%) had their data linked to CMS administrative claims for analyses. The median patient age of the patients was 82 years; 56% of patients were male, 85% of patients had NYHA functional class III or IV, and 93% of patients had grade 3 or greater MR. Postprocedure results were excellent: 92% of patients had grade 2 or less MR. In-hospital conversion to open surgery was infrequent (0.7%). In-hospital mortality was 2.7%, and major or life-threatening bleeding occurred in 3.9% of patients. Compared with the initial TVT registry report, the median length of stay decreased from 3 days to 2 days.

Follow-up was reported at 30 days and 1 year. The rates of mortality at 30 days and 1 year were

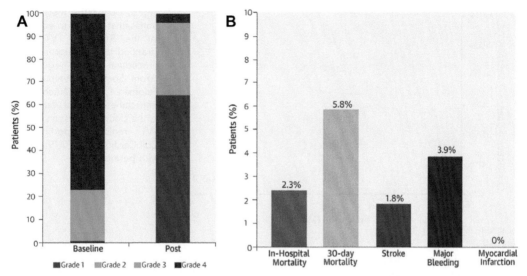

Fig. 3. (A) Change in the severity of mitral regurgitation and (B) 30-day adverse outcomes after transcatheter edge-to-edge repair in the STS/ACC TVT registry. (*From* Sorajja P, MacK M, Vemulapalli S, et al. Initial experience with commercial transcatheter mitral valve repair in the United States. J Am Coll Cardiol 2016;67(10):1129–40; with permission.)

25.2% and 25.8%, respectively; the rates of stroke were 1.4% at 30 days and 3.2% at 1 year; rehospitalization for heart failure within 1 year occurred in 20.2%. The cumulative rate of death or heart failure hospitalization at 1 year was 37.9%. On multivariate analysis, factors independently associated with 1-year mortality were increased age, lower LVEF, severe tricuspid regurgitation, dialysis, residual MR (>2+), and moderate to severe lung disease (Figs. 4–6).

The TVT registry reports illustrate that in the US commercial experience, patients undergoing transcatheter mitral valve are elderly with multiple comorbid conditions. Despite this, procedural success is high with low rates of in-hospital mortality. The longer-term mortality is not low, consistent with the high-risk characteristics of this cohort; specific subsets of patients, including those with substantial residual MR and significant tricuspid regurgitation, seem to have significantly worse outcomes. Incorporation of these poor prognostic factors may be important when considering selecting appropriate patients for the procedure. Furthermore, addressing these factors (eg, tricuspid repair)

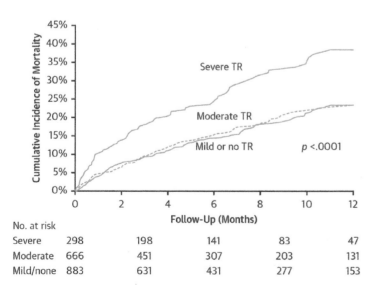

No. at risk

Severe	298	198	141	83	47
Moderate	666	451	307	203	131
Mild/none	883	631	431	277	153

Fig. 4. Cumulative mortality after transcatheter edge-to-edge repair in the STS/ACC TVT registry stratified by the severity of tricuspid regurgitation at baseline. TR, tricuspid regurgitation. (*From* Sorajja P, Vemulapalli S, Feldman T, et al. Outcomes with transcatheter mitral valve repair in the United States: an STS/ACC TVT registry report. J Am Coll Cardiol 2017;70(19):2315–27; with permission.)

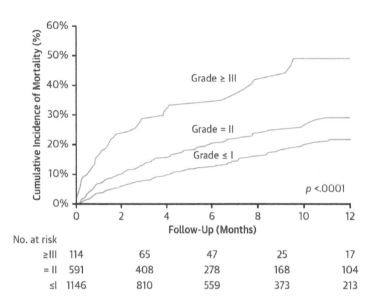

Fig. 5. Cumulative mortality after transcatheter edge-to-edge repair in the STS/ACC TVT registry stratified by the degree of post-procedural mitral regurgitation. (*From* Sorajja P, Vemulapalli S, Feldman T, et al. Outcomes with transcatheter mitral valve repair in the United States: an STS/ACC TVT registry report. J Am Coll Cardiol 2017;70(19):2315–27; with permission.)

could help improve long-term outcomes, although this must be evaluated in clinical trials.

EUROPEAN STUDIES

The MitraClip system received Conformité Européene (CE) mark approval in March 2008. Several European registries and observational studies have been performed since that time. Unlike the commercial experience in the United States, which is limited to patients with primary or mixed causes, the mechanism of MR in most patients undergoing transcatheter edge-to-edge repair in the European experience is functional: 60% to 70% of the studied population had functional MR and 30% to 40% had DMR.[11]

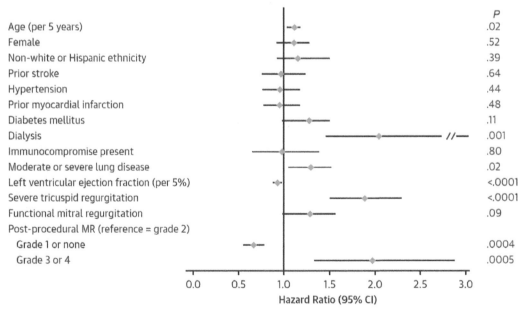

Fig. 6. Predictors of death or rehospitalization at 1 year after transcatheter edge-to-edge repair in TVT registry. CI, confidence interval. (*From* Sorajja P, Vemulapalli S, Feldman T, et al. Outcomes with transcatheter mitral valve repair in the United States: an STS/ACC TVT registry report. J Am Coll Cardiol 2017;70(19):2315–27; with permission.)

ACCESS-EU

The ACCESS-EU (ACCESS-Europe A Two-Phase Observational Study of the MitraClip System in Europe) study is a biphase, prospective, multi-center, nonrandomized, postapproval study of MitraClip across 14 European centers. The aim of the registry was to gain valuable information about this technology and its impact on health economics and clinical care. Preliminary 12-month results were published in 2013.[13,14] The study enrolled patients from April 2009 to April 2011. A total of 567 patients with 3+ or 4+ MR who were symptomatic or asymptomatic were included, 117 (20.1%) of whom had DMR. The mean age of patients with DMR was 75.6 years, 60% were more than 75 years of age, and 50% were male. Nearly three-quarters (73%) were NYHA functional class 3 or 4 and 113 (96.6%) had at least 3+ MR. Mitraclip implantation was successful in 111 of the 117 patients with DMR (94.9%). Mortality was 6% at 6 months and 17.1% at 12 months. The severity of the residual MR was less than or equal to 2+ in 88.7%, 77.7%, and 74.6% of patients at discharge, 6 months, and 12 months. With respect to heart failure symptoms, 80.8% of the patients with DMR were in NYHA class I or II at 12-month follow-up.

Therefore, the ACCESS-EU registry results show that, in the early postapproval European experience, a minority of patients were treated for DMR; these patients were generally older with poor functional class, although younger than those in the US TVT registry experience. The procedure itself was broadly successful, and, at 1 year postprocedure, approximately three-quarters of the treated patients had moderate or less MR, and symptomatic improvement was seen in the overwhelming majority.

Transcatheter Mitral Valve Interventions Registry

The Transcatheter Mitral Valve Interventions (TRAMI) registry is a German investigator-initiated registry that assessed outcomes of patients undergoing MitraClip placement at German centers. The TRAMI registry prospectively enrolled 828 patients from August 2010 to July 2013. Findings of the TRAMI registry have been reported since 2012.[15–18]

The mean age of the patients was 76.0 years; 60% of the patients were male. The mechanism of MR was secondary (functional) in 70%; the analysis did not stratify outcomes by functional or DMR. With this caveat in mind, the study population and outcomes were similar to what was found in other trials and registries. NYHA functional class was III or IV in 89% of patients, and baseline MR was 3+ or more in 94%. There was only 1 intraprocedural death and in-hospital mortality was 2.2%. The stroke rate was 0.9% and risk of pericardial tamponade was 1.9%. Major complications occurred in 12.8%, mainly driven by major bleeding complications (overall rate, 7.0%). The rate of SLDA was 2% and there were no cases of clip embolization. Older and more frail patients tended to have more complications.[15]

One-year follow-up were available in 749 (90.5%) patients.[16] Mortality was 4.5% at 30 days and 20.3% at 1 year. Predictors of 1-year mortality were NYHA functional class IV, anemia, serum creatinine level greater than or equal to 1.5 mg/dL, peripheral artery disease, LVEF less than 30%, severe tricuspid regurgitation, and procedural failure. There were more people with NYHA III and IV functional class in the TRAMI registry compared with TVT registry, likely because of the higher proportion of patients with functional MR in the registry. Despite the differences in mechanism of MR reflected in the 2 registries, the predictors of mortality post-MitraClip that were identified by the TRAMI registry are generally consistent with those that were identified within the TVT registry.

Getting Reduction of Mitral Insufficiency Registry

The GRASP (Getting Reduction of Mitral Insufficiency by Percutaneous Clip Implantation) registry was a single-center study at the University of Catania, Italy, and included 117 patients with 3+ or more MR who were thought to be high surgical risk who underwent percutaneous edge-to-edge mitral valve repair with MitraClip. Patients were enrolled from August 2008 to October 2012.[19] Similar to the TRAMI registry, most (76%) patients had functional MR and the remaining 24% had DMR. In contrast with the TRAMI registry, reported outcomes were stratified by type of MR. The average age of the 28 patients with DMR was 73 years, 68% were men, and 82% were NYHA III or IV functional class. There were no in-hospital or 30-day adverse events in the DMR group. There were no cases of clip detachment or embolization in either group. Deterioration to MR greater than or equal to 3+ occurred in 4% at 30 days and 25% at 1 year.

Mitraclip Asia-Pacific Registry

The MitraClip Asia-Pacific Registry (MARS) is a multicenter, retrospective registry of 8 centers in Australia, China, Indonesia, Malaysia, and

Table 1
Summary of key trials and registries of transcatheter edge-to-edge repair for primary (degenerative) mitral regurgitation

Registry/Trial	Sites	Year	Number of Patients	Major Inclusion Criteria	Major Exclusion Criteria	Mean Age (y)	DMR (%)	In-hospital Death (%)	30-d Death (%)	1-y Death (%)	IH MR ≤2+ (%)	30 d MR ≤2+ (%)	1-y MR ≤2+ (%)
EVEREST I	United States and Canada; 11 sites	2003–2006	55	MR ≥3+. Symptomatic or asymptomatic patients. LVEF 30%–50% and/or LVESD 50–55 mm or LVEF 50%–60% and LVESD<45 mm or LVEF>60 and LVESD 45–50 mm. Candidate for mitral valve surgery, including cardiopulmonary bypass	LVEF <30% and/or LVESD >55 mm. Mitral valve orifice area <4.0 cm². Leaflet anatomy not suitable for percutaneous repair	71	100	0	0	1.8	—	83.3	71.8
EVEREST II	United States and Canada; 37 sites	2005–2008	279	MR ≥3+. Symptomatic with LVEF>25%, LVESD ≤ 55 mm or asymptomatic (with LVEF 25% to 60%, LVESD ≥ 40 mm, new-onset atrial fibrillation, PASP>50 mm Hg at rest or >60 mm Hg with exercise)	LVEF ≤ 25%, and/or LVESD >55 mm, mitral valve orifice area <4.0 cm², leaflet anatomy not suitable for percutaneous repair	67	51	—	—	6	—	—	79

EVEREST II High Risk Registry Study	United States and Canada; 25 sites	2007–2008	78	MR ≥ 3+, STS predicted mortality ≥12%, or deemed to be high-risk surgical candidate by cardiac surgeon because of presence of certain indications (porcelain aorta, mobile ascending aortic atheroma, postradiation mediastinum, previous mediastinitis, functional MR with EF<40%, reoperation with patent grafts, 2 or more prior chest surgeries, hepatic cirrhosis, 3+ of high STS risk factors of creatinine level >2.5 mg/dL or prior chest surgery or age >75 y or EF<35%)	LVEF ≤ 20% and/or LVESD >60 mm, mitral valve orifice area <4.0 cm^2, or leaflet anatomy not suitable for percutaneous repair	77	41	—	7.7	24.4	—	72.9	77.8
REALISM High Risk Continuous Access Registry	United States and Canada; 39 sites	2009–2013	628	Same as EVEREST II High Risk Registry	Same as EVEREST II High Risk Registry	77	—	—	—	—	—	86.1	51.8
REALISM Non–High Risk Continuous Access Registry	United States and Canada; 39 sites	2009–2011	271	Same as EVEREST II Trial	Same as EVEREST II Trial	74	—	—	—	—	—	88.2	60.1

(continued on next page)

Table 1
(continued)

Registry/Trial	Sites	Year	Number of Patients	Major Inclusion Criteria	Major Exclusion Criteria	Mean Age (y)	DMR (%)	In-hospital Death (%)	30-d Death (%)	1-y Death (%)	IH MR ≤2+ (%)	30 d MR ≤2+ (%)	1-y MR ≤2+ (%)
TVT Registry	United States; 61 sites	2013–2014	2952	Symptomatic severe (grade 3 or 4), primary (degenerative) mitral regurgitation in patients who are at prohibitive surgical risk (STS score ≥6% for mitral valve repair and ≥8% for mitral valve replacement or presence of comorbidities that portend heightened risk	—	82	94.8	2.7	5.2	25.8	93	—	—
ACCESS-EU	Europe; 14 sites	2009–2011	567	Symptomatic or asymptomatic patients with 3+ or 4+ MR who were deemed too high risk for surgery and underwent percutaneous repair	—	74	20.1	—	6[a]	17.1[a]	88.7[a]	—	74.6[a]
TRAMI	Germany; 20 sites	2010–2013	749[b]	Symptomatic or asymptomatic patients with 3+ or 4+ MR who were deemed too high risk for surgery and underwent percutaneous repair	—	76	30	—	4.5	20.3	97.8 (moderate or less)	—	—

GRASP	Italy; 1 site	2008–2012	117	Symptomatic or asymptomatic patients with 3+ or 4+ MR who were deemed too high risk for surgery and underwent percutaneous repair	—	73[a]	24	0	0.9	9.4	100[a]	96[a]	75[a]
Asia-Pacific Registry	Asia; 8 sites	2011–2013	163	Symptomatic or asymptomatic patients with 3+ or 4+ MR who were deemed too high risk for surgery and underwent percutaneous repair	—	71	46	4[a]	6.7[a]	—	92[a]	77	—
MitraSwiss Registry	Switzerland; 4 sites	2009–2011	155	Symptomatic or asymptomatic patients with 3+ or 4+ MR who were deemed too high risk for surgery and underwent percutaneous repair	—	77	38	4	4	10	85	—	61[c]

Abbreviations: EF, ejection fraction; PASP, systolic PA-pressure

[a] Rates for patients with DMR only; if DMR-only data not available, rates are for all MR (functional MR and DMR).

[b] Prospective cohort.

[c] Follow-up at 6 months.

Singapore.[20,21] In the initial report,[20] 142 patients were enrolled encompassing the period between February 2011 and October 2013. Of these patients, 46% had DMR. Acute procedural success was 93.7%. At 30-day follow-up, 76.8% had less than or equal to 2+ MR. A second report stratified the results of the outcomes by MR mechanism.[21] A total of 163 patients underwent MitraClip placement; 88 of whom (54%) had functional MR and 75 of whom (46%) had DMR. The average age of the patients with DMR was 72.7 years, 64% were men, 58% of patients had NYHA functional class III or IV symptoms, and 82.7% had 4+ MR. Acute procedural success, defined as immediate reduction of MR to less than or equal to 2+, was 92% in the DMR cohort. SLDA occurred in 4 patients (5%). At 30 days, the mortality was 6.7% (5 out of 75). Major adverse events occurred in 14.7% (11 out of 75), comprising death (5 out of 11), transfusion of greater than or equal to 2 units of blood (2 out of 11), sepsis (2 out of 11), open mitral valve surgery (1 out of 11), and prolonged intubation (1 out of 11). Functional class was improved by the procedure, with 83% of patients being NYHA functional class I to II at 30 days. There was also significant improvement in LV dimensions at 30 days.

MitraSwiss Registry

The MitraSwiss registry included 4 cardiac centers in Switzerland.[22,23] The outcomes of the first 100 patients undergoing a MitraClip procedure from February 2009 to April 2011 were included in the initial report.[22] Of these 100 patients, the mechanism of MR was degenerative in 38. The average age of the study population was 77 years, 67% were male, 70% had 4+ MR, and 82% were NYHA functional class III or IV. Acute procedural success in the DMR group was 92% and there were no in-hospital deaths. Two-year follow-up was available in 74 patients, of whom 28 were part of the DMR group.[23] Of these patients, 93% had less than or equal to 2+ MR. For the overall cohort, mortalities at 1 and 2 years were 19% and 25%. The degree of residual MR correlated with cumulative survival.

SUMMARY

The registries and trials of percutaneous mitral valve repair for DMR provide important insight into the safety and efficacy of transcatheter edge-to-edge mitral valve repair with the MitraClip (Table 1). Acute procedural success has improved as operators have gained more experience. The procedure has an excellent safety profile: in the large, commercial experience described by the TVT registry, the rate of in-hospital mortality was only 2.7% despite the extremely high-risk cohort as reflected by age, comorbidities, and STS-PROM scores. MR severity at 1 year postprocedure seems to be less than or equal to 2+ in approximately three-quarters of patients, with favorable outcomes in terms of reduction in heart failure hospitalizations, NYHA functional class, and LV dimensions. Findings from the EVEREST High Risk Cohort show that these results are durable. Transcatheter edge-to-edge mitral valve repair seems superior to medical therapy, although these comparisons are limited by study design and power. Registry data have helped define key predictors of poor outcomes postprocedure, including the importance of a reduction in MR to at least 2+ or less. Further long-term follow-up results from these registries will continue to provide valuable information with regard to efficacy, durability, and patient selection for percutaneous edge-to-edge repair for DMR.

REFERENCES

1. Summary of safety and effectiveness data (SSED) for MitraClip® Clip Delivery System. Available at: https://www.accessdata.fda.gov/cdrh_docs/pdf10/P100009B.pdf. Accessed November 7, 2018.

2. Feldman T, Wasserman HS, Herrmann HC, et al. Percutaneous mitral valve repair using the edge-to-edge technique: six-month results of the EVEREST phase I clinical trial. J Am Coll Cardiol 2005; 46(11):2134–40.

3. Feldman T, Kar S, Rinaldi M, et al. Percutaneous mitral repair with the Mitraclip system. safety and midterm durability in the initial EVEREST (Endovascular Valve Edge-to-Edge REpair Study) Cohort. J Am Coll Cardiol 2009;54(8):686–94.

4. Feldman T, Foster E, Glower DD, et al. Percutaneous repair or surgery for mitral regurgitation. N Engl J Med 2011;364(15):1395–406.

5. Mauri L, Foster E, Glower DD, et al. 4-Year results of a randomized controlled trial of percutaneous repair versus surgery for mitral regurgitation. J Am Coll Cardiol 2013;62(4):317–28.

6. Feldman T, Kar S, Elmariah S, et al. Randomized comparison of percutaneous repair and surgery for mitral regurgitation 5-year results of EVEREST II. J Am Coll Cardiol 2015;66(25): 2844–54.

7. Whitlow PL, Feldman T, Pedersen WR, et al. Acute and 12-month results with catheter-based mitral valve leaflet repair: the EVEREST II (Endovascular Valve Edge-to-Edge Repair) high risk study. J Am Coll Cardiol 2012;59(2):130–9.

8. Kar S, Feldman T, Qasim A, et al. Five-year outcomes of transcatheter reduction of significant mitral regurgitation in high-surgical-risk patients. Heart 2018;2(3) [pii: heartjnl-2017-312605].

9. Real World Expanded Multicenter Study of the MitraClip® System (REALISM). Available at: https://clinicaltrials.gov/ct2/show/results/NCT01931956. Accessed November 7, 2018.

10. Lim DS, Reynolds MR, Feldman T, et al. Improved functional status and quality of life in prohibitive surgical risk patients with degenerative mitral regurgitation after transcatheter mitral valve repair. J Am Coll Cardiol 2014;64(2):182–92.

11. Sorajja P, MacK M, Vemulapalli S, et al. Initial experience with commercial transcatheter mitral valve repair in the United States. J Am Coll Cardiol 2016;67(10):1129–40.

12. Sorajja P, Vemulapalli S, Feldman T, et al. Outcomes with transcatheter mitral valve repair in the United States: An STS/ACC TVT registry report. J Am Coll Cardiol 2017;70(19):2315–27.

13. Maisano F, Franzen O, Baldus S, et al. Percutaneous mitral valve interventions in the real world: early and 1-year results from the ACCESS-EU, a prospective, multicenter, nonrandomized post-approval study of the Mitraclip therapy in Europe. J Am Coll Cardiol 2013;62(12):1052–61.

14. Reichenspurner H, Schillinger W, Baldus S, et al. Clinical outcomes through 12 months in patients with degenerative mitral regurgitation treated with the Mitraclip® device in the ACCESS-EUrope phase I trial. Eur J Cardiothorac Surg 2013;44(4):e280–8.

15. Eggebrecht H, Schelle S, Puls M, et al. Risk and outcomes of complications during and after MitraClip implantation: Experience in 828 patients from the German TRAnscatheter mitral valve interventions (TRAMI) registry. Catheter Cardiovasc Interv 2015;86(4):728–35.

16. Puls M, Lubos E, Boekstegers P, et al. One-year outcomes and predictors of mortality after MitraClip therapy in contemporary clinical practice: results from the German transcatheter mitral valve interventions registry. Eur Heart J 2016;37(8):703–12.

17. Eggebrecht H, Mehta RH, Lubos E, et al. MitraClip in high- versus low-volume centers: an analysis from the German TRAMI registry. JACC Cardiovasc Interv 2018;11(3):287–97.

18. Kalbacher D, Schäfer U, V Bardeleben RS, et al. Long-term outcome, survival and predictors of mortality after MitraClip therapy: Results from the German Transcatheter Mitral Valve Interventions (TRAMI) registry. Int J Cardiol 2018. https://doi.org/10.1016/j.ijcard.2018.08.023.

19. Grasso C, Capodanno D, Scandura S, et al. One- and twelve-month safety and efficacy outcomes of patients undergoing edge-to-edge percutaneous mitral valve repair (from the grasp registry). Am J Cardiol 2013;111(10):1482–7.

20. Yeo KK, Yap J, Yamen E, et al. Percutaneous mitral valve repair with the MitraClip: early results from the MitraClip Asia-Pacific Registry (MARS). EuroIntervention 2014;10(5):620–5.

21. Tay E, Muda N, Yap J, et al. The MitraClip Asia-Pacific registry: Differences in outcomes between functional and degenerative mitral regurgitation. Catheter Cardiovasc Interv 2016;87(7):E275–81.

22. Sürder D, Pedrazzini G, Gaemperli O, et al. Predictors for efficacy of percutaneous mitral valve repair using the MitraClip system: the results of the MitraSwiss registry. Heart 2013;99(14):1034–40.

23. Toggweiler S, Zuber M, Sürder D, et al. Two-year outcomes after percutaneous mitral valve repair with the MitraClip system: Durability of the procedure and predictors of outcome. Open Heart 2014;1(1). https://doi.org/10.1136/openhrt-2014-000056.

Transcatheter Mitral Valve Direct Annuloplasty with the Millipede IRIS Ring

Jason H. Rogers, MD[a],*, Walter D. Boyd, MD[b],
Thomas W. Smith, MD[a], Steven F. Bolling, MD[c]

KEYWORDS

• Mitral regurgitation • Transcatheter mitral valve repair • Mitral annuloplasty • Transcatheter ring

KEY POINTS

• Mitral valve ring annuloplasty is a surgical gold standard and is used routinely during surgical mitral valve repair of primary or secondary mitral regurgitation.
• The Millipede IRIS annuloplasty ring is the first transcatheter, transfemoral, transseptal, semirigid, complete annuloplasty ring to be delivered to the mitral valve annulus.
• Initial results in humans demonstrate that the Millipede IRIS ring is safe, and can effectively reduce the mitral annular diameter leading to a clinically significant reduction or elimination of mitral regurgitation.

INTRODUCTION

In the nearly 50 years since mitral valve annuloplasty was introduced as a groundbreaking technique for mitral valve reconstruction, annuloplasty has become a standard part of successful surgical mitral valve (MV) repair.[1] Chronic mitral regurgitation (MR) is frequently associated with structural heart changes, including left atrial (LA) and left ventricular (LV) enlargement, which lead to dilation of the mitral annulus. This dilation causes and contributes to MR progression in patients with chronic disease. Surgery for primary MR repairs leaflet abnormalities (such as MV prolapse) that cause the valvular dysfunction. Repair includes plication or resection of the leaflets, and/or chordal replacement when indicated. Surgical repair is more effective and more durable when an annuloplasty ring is added, so this has become routine for primary MR correction. In contrast, secondary MR begins with LV dysfunction, which causes enlargement

of the mitral annulus and apical tethering of the MV leaflets. These disrupt proper coaptation during systole. By itself, mitral ring annuloplasty can correct secondary MR in patients who do not have excessive LV size or leaflet tethering.

Ideally in the foreseeable future, enough techniques will be developed for transcatheter MV repair to match the effectiveness and durability of surgical correction. Transcatheter approaches will offer an entirely new option for the many patients with MR whose comorbidities disqualify them for surgery due to the high risk.[2] Herein, we report on the mechanism of action, technique, and outcomes of the first successful transcatheter transfemoral annuloplasty treatment of MR using the Millipede IRIS semirigid complete annular reshaping ring.

THE MILLIPEDE IRIS DEVICE

The Millipede IRIS annuloplasty ring (Millipede, Inc., Santa Rosa, CA) is a semirigid, complete

---

Disclosures: Drs S.F. Bolling, W.D. Boyd, J.H. Rogers, and T.W. Smith are consultants to Millipede, Inc.
[a] Division of Cardiovascular Medicine, University of California, Davis Medical Center, 4860 Y Street, Suite 2820, Sacramento, CA 95817, USA; [b] Division of Cardiothoracic Surgery, University of California, Davis Medical Center, 2221 Stockton Boulevard, Suite 2112, Sacramento, CA 95817, USA; [c] Department of Cardiac Surgery, University of Michigan Health System, Floor 3 Reception C, 1500 E Medical Center Dr SPC 5856, Ann Arbor, MI 48109-5856, USA
* Corresponding author.
E-mail address: jhrogers@ucdavis.edu

(closed) ring manufactured from laser-cut and heat-set nickel-titanium alloy (nitinol). Eight helical stainless-steel anchors are preattached to the base of the ring. Each anchor rotates independently and attaches directly to the mitral annulus. If the operator is not satisfied with initial placement, each anchor can be retracted or "unscrewed," moved, and redeployed. The upper part of the device has 8 sliding collars. These also can be manipulated individually. When put under tension, each collar draws the 2 adjacent helical anchors closer together (Fig. 1). Because each collar shortens the linked portion of the ring, operators can customize the final annular circumference and diameter. Annuloplasty can be targeted to the most dilated portions of the annulus by judiciously tightening individual crowns. The IRIS procedure consists of 3 basic steps: (1) placement, (2) anchoring, and (3) actuation (Fig. 2). The device has been designed to allow repositioning and retrieval until the IRIS ring has been fully released from the delivery system.

IMPLANTATION PROCEDURE

A report of the first-in-human experience with the Millipede IRIS device was published in 2018.[3] In this report, we used the following inclusion criteria to enroll patients for treatment with the IRIS device: (1) 3 or 4+ ischemic or nonischemic predominantly secondary MR with a dilated mitral annulus; (2) symptomatic New York Heart Association (NYHA) class II, III, or ambulatory IV; (3) LV end-systolic diameter ≤65 mm; (4) surgical MV correction was a viable option. Exclusion criteria for this initial series were as follows: (1) LV ejection fraction <20%; (2) untreated significant CAD or any revascularization within 30 days; (3) aortic valve disease requiring intervention; (4) pulmonary artery systolic pressure >70 mm Hg; (5) right-sided congestive heart failure; (6) any prior mitral or tricuspid valve surgery; (7) active infection or life expectancy <12 months. Mitral annular dimensions were measured by transthoracic and transesophageal echocardiography, and MR quantification was performed using the Mitral Valve Academic Research Consortium criteria.[4] Preprocedure and postprocedure LA and LV diastolic volumes were measured using gated cardiac computed tomography scans (Clinical Imaging Analytics, Guerneville, CA). Initial follow-up was performed at 30 days, with additional follow-up planned for 6 months and 1 year.

SURGICAL IMPLANTS

Before transcatheter delivery of the Millipede IRIS, the first human implants were performed surgically using median sternotomy, standard bicaval cannulation, and cardiopulmonary bypass. These surgical implants (referred to as Phase 1) established the safety and efficacy of the ring. Using a short catheter, the device was placed onto the mitral annulus. Each helical anchor was screwed into the tissue under direct vision (Fig. 3). The collars were then rotated to actuate the device and reduce the mitral diameter until no MR was present by surgical "bulb irrigation" testing with saline. Three of these temporary implants were performed before planned surgical annuloplasty. Subsequently, 4 patients were treated with permanent implants in both the mitral (n = 4) and mitral + tricuspid (n = 2) position.

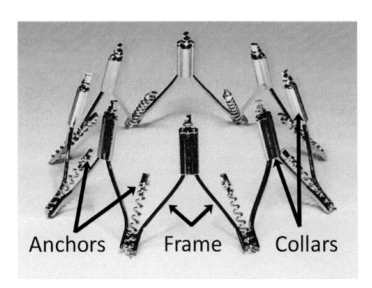

Anchors   Frame   Collars

Fig. 1. The transcatheter Millipede IRIS device. The Millipede IRIS device consists of a nitinol frame, 8 helical anchors that attach to the mitral annulus, and 8 sliding collars that allow actuation of the device and reduction of the mitral annular diameter. (Image provided courtesy of Boston Scientific. © 2019 Boston Scientific Corporation or its affiliates. All rights reserved.)

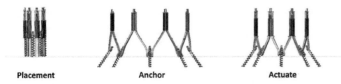

Placement   Anchor   Actuate

In Phase 2 of the Millipede IRIS first-in-human series, we delivered a lower-profile transcatheter IRIS ring to the mitral annulus using a transfemoral, transseptal transcatheter approach (Fig. 4). These procedures were performed under general anesthesia in the cardiac catheterization laboratory. Right femoral vein access was obtained and preclosed with two 6-French Proglide devices (Abbott, Santa Clara, CA). Transseptal puncture was performed in the superior and posterior portion of the interatrial septum using standard techniques at a height of ~4 cm above the plane of the mitral annulus. The IRIS deflectable guide catheter was advanced from the right femoral vein, across the septum, and into the left atrium over a 0.035-inch wire. The guide was aspirated and flushed, and heparin was given to maintain an activated clotting time of 250 to 300 seconds. Next, the IRIS device, which was preloaded onto the 24-French deflectable IRIS delivery catheter, was advanced through the guide catheter. Under fluoroscopic and echocardiographic guidance, we directed the IRIS device to a position superior to the annulus and centered over the mitral orifice. The device was expanded and anchored on the mitral annulus using both transesophageal echocardiography (TEE) and intracardiac echocardiography (ICE). ICE allows direct visualization of each individual anchor attachment in an optimal location on the mitral annulus. The IRIS device was then actuated to achieve the desired reduction in the mitral annular diameter. After confirming circumflex coronary patency by angiography, the IRIS device was released from the delivery catheter. The delivery catheter was then removed, followed by removal of the guide catheter. To simplify later analysis, we chose to close all iatrogenic atrial septal defects (iASDs) in the first 3 transcatheter cases with 10 mm Amplatzer septal occluders (Abbott, Santa Clara, CA). The femoral vein was closed with the previously deployed Proglides.

CLINICAL RESULTS

In our initial clinical report, 7 patients received the IRIS ring in Phase 1 (n = 4) and Phase 2 (n = 3). The average age of the patients treated was 60.3 years. The local heart team managed appropriate medical therapy. All patients were candidates for surgical MV annuloplasty. The 4 Phase 1 patients received the IRIS ring through a conventional open surgical approach. The subsequent 3 patients in Phase 2 received the transcatheter mitral IRIS rings to the mitral annulus, and their average left ventricular ejection fraction (LVEF) was 42% ± 19%. There was no device-related procedural death, stroke, or myocardial infarction.

In all of the patients who received the IRIS device, the preprocedure mitral septolateral (SL) diameter as determined by transthoracic

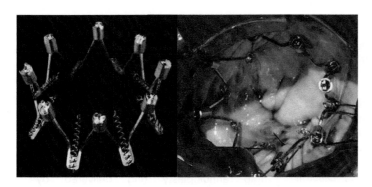

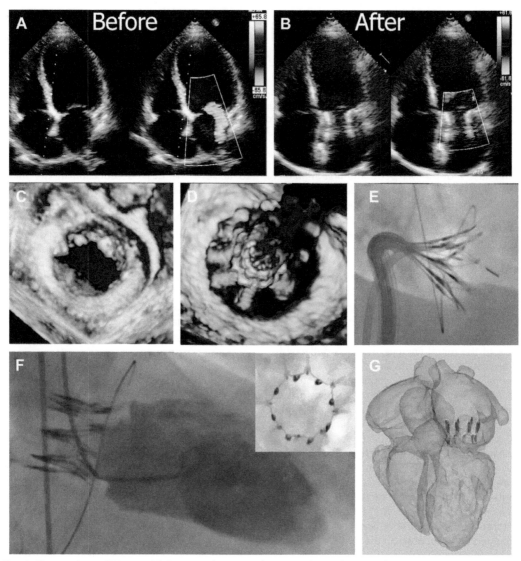

Fig. 4. Transcatheter IRIS ring. (*A*) Preprocedure transthoracic echocardiogram showing 3+ secondary MR. (*B*) Thirty-day post-IRIS implantation with no MR. (*C*) Baseline native MV annulus on TEE. (*D*) Centering the IRIS ring on the MV before full expansion and anchoring. (*E*) Fluoroscopic appearance of transfemoral transseptal delivery of IRIS ring. (*F*) Final fluoroscopic appearance during left ventriculogram and en face view (inset). (*G*) Computed tomography scan at 30 days showing position of IRIS ring (*blue*) in the heart. (*From* Rogers JH, Boyd WD, Smith TW, et al. Transcatheter annuloplasty for mitral regurgitation with an adjustable semi-rigid complete ring: initial experience with the Millipede IRIS device. Structural Heart. 2018;2(1):43–50; with permission.)

echocardiography (TTE) was reduced from a baseline of 38.0 ± 4.1 mm to 25.9 ± 4.9 mm at 30 days. This is an average SL reduction of 31.8% (**Fig. 5**).

Every patient in the study demonstrated reduction of MR, with all patients showing a decline from a baseline of 3 or 4+ MR to 0 or 1+ MR at 30 days (**Fig. 6**). We observed improvements in NYHA Class (**Fig. 7**), and reductions in LV diastolic volumes (**Fig. 8**). Diastolic

LV volumes decreased from 182.4 ± 54.3 mL, to 115.3 ± 98.8 mL at 30 days (36.8% reduction; n = 7). The LA volume was 172.7 ± 67.2 mL at baseline and 133.6 ± 62.3 mL at 30 days (n = 7).

DISCUSSION

The Millipede IRIS ring is the first complete semi-rigid annuloplasty ring delivered by a

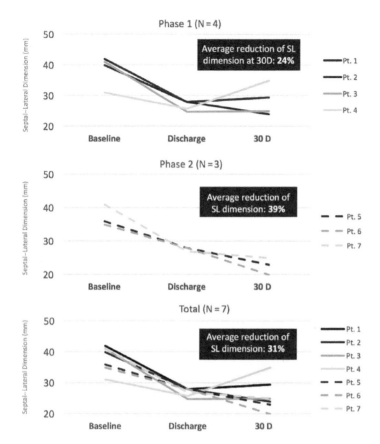

Fig. 5. Reduction in septal-lateral dimension. Phase 1, surgical implants. Phase 2, transcatheter implants. (*From* Rogers JH, Boyd WD, Smith TW, et al. Transcatheter annuloplasty for mitral regurgitation with an adjustable semi-rigid complete ring: initial experience with the Millipede IRIS device. Structural Heart 2018;2(1):43–50; with permission.)

percutaneous, transfemoral, and transseptal route. The IRIS ring operates by complete and circumferential annuloplasty. Initial patients showed reductions in the mitral SL diameter, MR, LV volumes, and improvement in NYHA Class.

Mitral annuloplasty is used frequently during surgical MV correction and presently is part of the "gold standard" of successful repair. Annuloplasty is routinely applied in 2 patient subgroups. In restrictive annuloplasty, an undersized ring is used to normalize the anterior-posterior mitral annular diameter. This can be a stand-alone therapy for secondary MR. In the second subgroup, annuloplasty rings have been used to stabilize the annulus in repair of primary MR. This has been shown to significantly improve the durability of surgical repair.[5]

Data from earlier studies show that complete (closed) rigid annuloplasty rings have less MR recurrence over time than partial (open) flexible bands. Spoor and colleagues[6] retrospectively reviewed outcomes in 289 patients with LVEF ≤30% who received an undersized complete mitral annuloplasty ring for MV repair in the setting of ischemic or idiopathic cardiomyopathy. A total of 170 patients had a flexible complete ring and 119 patients received a 26-mm or 28-mm undersized nonflexible complete ring. In the flexible group, 9.4% required a repeat procedure because of significant recurrent MR (average time to reoperation 2.4 years), compared with only 2.5% in the nonflexible group (average time to reoperation 4.0 years).

Millipede's IRIS offers a mode of action and function that is unique among transcatheter devices at this time. The device is a semirigid complete ring that attaches directly to the entire mitral annulus and can normalize the mitral anterior-posterior diameter in properly selected patients. The device is supra-annular and does not interfere with the LV outflow tract. It has previously been shown that normalization of the SL diameter is one of the most important effects in restoring leaflet coaptation and abolishing ischemic MR.[7] In our clinical experience thus far, the Millipede IRIS system has effectively normalized the SL diameter of the mitral annulus. As stated previously, we observed a

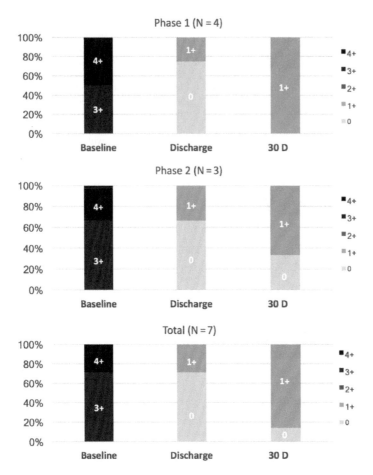

Fig. 6. MR grade. Reproduced with permission. Phase 1, surgical implants. Phase 2, transcatheter implants. (*From* Rogers JH, Boyd WD, Smith TW, et al. Transcatheter annuloplasty for mitral regurgitation with an adjustable semi-rigid complete ring: initial experience with the Millipede IRIS device. Structural Heart 2018;2(1):43–50; with permission.)

reduction in average mitral SL diameter from 38.0 to 25.9 mm, on average, 31.8%.[3] Although we closed the iASDs in this early series, in future studies the iASD can likely be left alone without closure as with many other transseptal therapies.

The Millipede IRIS ring also can be used in conjunction with transcatheter edge-to-edge repair effected by the MitraClip device.[8] Furthermore, we envision the possibility of the IRIS ring serving as a "docking station" for subsequent transcatheter MV in ring implantation.

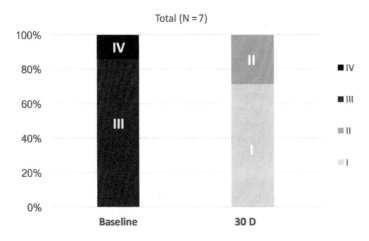

Fig. 7. NYHA functional class. (*From* Rogers JH, Boyd WD, Smith TW, et al. Transcatheter annuloplasty for mitral regurgitation with an adjustable semi-rigid complete ring: initial experience with the Millipede IRIS device. Structural Heart 2018;2(1):43–50; with permission.)

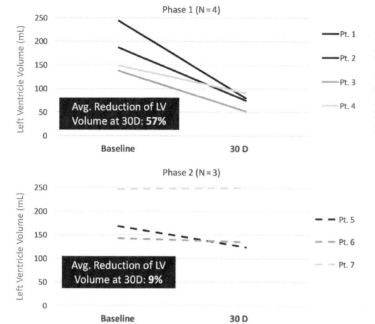

Fig. 8. Reduction in LV volume. Phase 1, surgical implants. Phase 2, transcatheter implants. (*From* Rogers JH, Boyd WD, Smith TW, et al. Transcatheter annuloplasty for mitral regurgitation with an adjustable semi-rigid complete ring: initial experience with the Millipede IRIS device. Structural Heart 2018;2(1):43–50; with permission.)

SUMMARY

The Millipede IRIS mitral annuloplasty ring is the first transcatheter complete semirigid ring to be delivered to the mitral annulus through a transfemoral, transseptal approach. We are actively pursuing improvements in the device, delivery system, and intraprocedural imaging. Ongoing clinical trials of the device will yield additional information.

REFERENCES

1. Carpentier A. Reconstructive valvuloplasty. A new technique of mitral valvuloplasty. Presse Med 1969; 77(7):251–3 [in French].
2. Iung B, Baron G, Butchart EG, et al. A prospective survey of patients' with valvular heart disease in Europe: The Euro Heart Survey on Valvular Heart Disease. Eur Heart J 2003;24(13):1231–43.
3. Rogers JH, Boyd WD, Smith TW, et al. Transcatheter annuloplasty for mitral regurgitation with an adjustable semi-rigid complete ring: initial experience with the millipede IRIS device. Structural Heart 2018;2(1):43–50.
4. Stone GW, Vahanian AS, Adams DH, et al. Clinical trial design principles and endpoint definitions for transcatheter mitral valve repair and replacement: part 1: clinical trial design principles: a consensus document from the mitral valve academic research consortium. J Am Coll Cardiol 2015;66(3):278–307.
5. Gillinov AM, Cosgrove DM, Blackstone EH, et al. Durability of mitral valve repair for degenerative disease. J Thorac Cardiovasc Surg 1998;116(5):734–43.
6. Spoor MT, Geltz A, Bolling SF. Flexible versus nonflexible mitral valve rings for congestive heart failure: differential durability of repair. Circulation 2006; 114(1 Suppl):I67–71.
7. Timek TA, Lai DT, Tibayan F, et al. Septal-lateral annular cinching abolishes acute ischemic mitral regurgitation. J Thorac Cardiovasc Surg 2002; 123(5):881–8.
8. Rogers JH, Boyd WD, Smith TWR, et al. Combined mitraclip edge-to-edge repair with millipede iris mitral annuloplasty. JACC Cardiovasc Interv 2018; 11(3):323–4.

Left Ventricular Outflow Tract Obstruction
A Potential Obstacle for Transcatheter Mitral Valve Therapy

Jeremy Ben-Shoshan, MD[a,b], Dee Dee Wang, MD[c],
Anita W. Asgar, MD, MSc[a,b],*

KEYWORDS

- Transcatheter mitral intervention • Left ventricular outflow tract obstruction
- Mitral valve disease

KEY POINTS

- Left ventricular outflow tract (LVOT) obstruction is a complex interplay of anatomic, dynamic, and mechanical factors and may occur after surgical or transcatheter intervention.
- Adequate imaging evaluation with computed tomography and echocardiography is essential before transcatheter mitral intervention to assess the risk of LVOT obstruction.
- There are several experimental therapeutic options for LVOT obstruction post–transcatheter mitral valve replacement, but to date outcomes remain suboptimal; prediction and preemptive therapy may be a more promising option.

INTRODUCTION

Transcatheter mitral valve replacement (TMVR) is emerging as a promising therapeutic option for patients with mitral valve disease, in particular for those at high surgical risk. Clinical data accumulated thus far have demonstrated the complexity and challenges of this new intervention. A recognized potential complication of TMVR is obstruction of the left ventricular outflow tract (LVOT) by the new valve prosthesis. In the current review, the authors summarize the known mechanisms of LVOT obstruction following mitral valve intervention, describe pre-TMVR imaging for prediction of iatrogenic LVOT obstruction, and discuss potential therapeutic options if it should occur.

LEFT VENTRICULAR OUTFLOW TRACT OBSTRUCTION FOLLOWING MITRAL VALVE SURGERY
Surgical Mitral Valve Repair

LVOT obstruction following mitral valve intervention was first described by Termini and colleagues[1] in 1977 following surgical mitral valve repair. They reported systolic anterior motion (SAM) of the mitral valve apparatus accompanied by a paradoxic motion of the interventricular septum, resulting in narrowing of the aortomitral angle and dynamic LVOT obstruction.[1] Kreindel and colleagues[2] later described the development of SAM after semirigid ring insertion, caused by the Venturi effect, in which the pressure drop with systolic emptying pulls a redundant anterior mitral leaflet (AML) toward the LVOT (see **Fig. 2**). Milhaneau and

---

[a] Department of Medicine, Montreal Heart Institute, Montreal, Quebec, Canada; [b] Université de Montréal, 5000 rue Belanger, Montreal, Quebec H1T1C8, Canada; [c] Center for Structural Heart Disease, Henry Ford Health System, 2799 West Grand Boulevard, Detroit, MI 48202, USA
* Corresponding author. Montreal Heart Institute, 5000 Belanger Street, Montreal, Quebec H1T 1C8, Canada.
E-mail address: anita.asgar@umontreal.ca

Intervent Cardiol Clin 8 (2019) 269–278
https://doi.org/10.1016/j.iccl.2019.02.009
2211-7458/19/© 2019 Elsevier Inc. All rights reserved.

colleagues[3] described an LVOT obstruction prevalence of 4% to 5% following mitral valve repair that reached 14% in patients with "high-risk" anatomic factors: mitral valve insufficiency of degenerative origin with excess leaflet tissue, a nondilated left ventricular cavity, and a narrow aortomitral angle. Later, echocardiographic studies in patients undergoing mitral valve repair demonstrated an anterior displacement of the coaptation point toward the LVOT caused by redundant mitral leaflets.[4] As a result, leaflet coaptation of the AML and posterior mitral leaflets (PML) occurs more at the base of the AML with more leaflet slack close to the LVOT with potential for obstruction. In fact, the "sliding leaflet" surgical technique developed by Carpentier consisted of reduction of the height of the PML and efficiently lowered the occurrence of LVOT obstruction following mitral valve repair.[5]

In a small study in patients with myxomatous mitral valve disease undergoing surgical repair, SAM/LVOT obstruction was found to be associated with a relatively lower AML/PML length ratio, as assessed preoperatively by transesophageal echocardiography.[6] Based on their findings, the investigators suggested a greater reduction in the posterior leaflet height during surgery, if the above ratio is 1.3 or lower, particularly if the distance from the coaptation point to the septum is 2.5 cm or less.[6] In a more recent echocardiography study by Varghese and colleagues,[7] independent predictors of developing SAM after surgical mitral valve repair were a small left ventricle (end diastolic diameter <45 mm), tall posterior leaflet height (>15 mm), a narrow angle between the planes of the aortic and mitral annulus (<120°), a short coaptation-septum distance (<25 mm), and an enlarged basal septal diameter (≥15 mm). The investigators suggested that the above parameters might guide the operators to consider appropriate measures to minimize the risk of LVOT obstruction, such as an upsized ring, ensuring a postrepair posterior leaflet height less than 15 mm and avoiding inotropes on weaning from bypass.[7]

Surgical Mitral Valve Replacement

LVOT obstruction has also been described following surgical mitral valve replacement.[8–10] Anatomically, the aortic and mitral valves are in fibrous continuity (Fig. 1); therefore, placement of a prosthetic valve in the mitral annulus might result in projection of the prosthesis into the left ventricular cavity in close proximity to the aortic annulus.[8,10] In addition, preoperative redundancy of the chordal apparatus, such as mitral regurgitation secondary to mitral valve prolapse, coupled with decreased chordal support following surgery, can contribute to SAM of the AML remnants after mitral valve replacement with preservation of the valve leaflets.[11] Of note, the decrease in left ventricular volume overload following resolution of mitral regurgitation may itself cause a reduction in LVOT area. This further reduction in the circumference of the LVOT induced by the traction of the prosthesis tightly sutured to the MV annulus, particularly with small devices (30 and smaller), may further increase the potential of LVOT obstruction.[12]

TRANSCATHETER MITRAL VALVE REPLACEMENT AND LEFT VENTRICULAR OUTFLOW TRACT OBSTRUCTION
Pathophysiology of Left Ventricular Outflow Tract Obstruction after Transcatheter Mitral Valve Replacement

LVOT obstruction is a known complication of TMVR. TMVR in mitral annulus calcification (MAC) has the highest associated rate of LVOTO, followed by TMVR in degenerative ring (valve-in-ring [ViR]), then TMVR valve-in-valve (ViV). The mechanisms of obstruction are similar to those previously discussed with surgical mitral repair and replacement, although with certain distinctions (Table 1).[13] Insertion of transcatheter heart valve (THV) into the mitral valve apparatus compresses the existing LVOT area, whereas the "native" portion of the LVOT, confined to the basal septum and intervalvular fibrosa, remains mostly unchanged.[14,15]

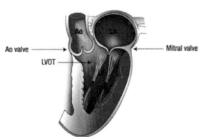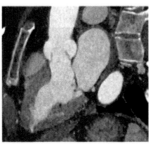

Fig. 1. Mitral valve with corresponding computed tomographic reconstructed image.

Table 1		
Factors contributing to LVOT obstruction following transcatheter mitral valve replacement		
Anatomic Factors	**Dynamic Factors**	**Mechanical Factors**
1. Small predicted neo-LVOT ($<=189.4$ mm^2) 2. Redundancy of the anterior mitral leaflet 3. Small LV cavity 4. Hypertrophic cardiomyopathy 5. Septal hypertrophy or asymmetric septal hypertrophy 6. Chordal redundancy 7. Mitral annular calcification 8. Aortomitral angle	1. Hypercontractile LV 2. Atrial fibrillation 3. Volume status/loading conditions 4. Hypertrophic cardiomyopathy 5. Left ventricular remodeling	1. Flaring of transcatheter devices placed in the mitral position 2. Extreme ventricular deployment of transcatheter heart valve 3. Interaction with aortic prosthesis

Abbreviation: LV, left ventricular.

This compressed and remodeled "neo-LVOT" is delineated anteriorly by the patient's native AML in ViR and valve-in-MAC TMVR. In TMVR ViV, the most anterior frame of the bioprosthetic device impinges on the neo-LVOT. Implantation of the transcatheter heart valve in a bioprosthesis results in opening of the leaflets of the surgical bioprosthesis, which are then pinned open by the stent of the transcatheter heart valve toward the LVOT, potentially resulting in a fixed systolic LVOT obstruction, resulting in a phenomenon known as "permanent anterior motion" of the bioprosthetic leaflet.[16–18]

Mechanical factors at the time of TMVR deployment also contribute to the added risk of LVOTO during the procedure. In an effort to minimize the risk of device embolization, structural operators inherently oversize transcatheter heart valves for the mitral position and flare the transcatheter heart valve to promote valve anchoring.[14,15,19] In ViV TMVR, an understanding of the bioprosthetic leaflet architecture also helps in prediction modeling for LVOTO. Bench studies have shown that bovine pericardial leaflets do not crinkle during ViV procedures. In contrast, porcine leaflets stand tall and may result in more significant LVOT obstruction.[20] Key to successful TMVR is an understanding of the risk factors for LVOTO known for decades by mitral surgeons after surgical mitral valve replacements, as well as left ventricular cavity size, septal hypertrophy,[21] and aortomitral angle that are more dangerous in the transcatheter world, where device placement cannot be manipulated postimplantation.

Incidence of Left Ventricular Outflow Tract Obstruction

In a multicenter retrospective study evaluating TMVR outcomes in patients with severe MAC

(n = 64), Guerrero and colleagues[19] reported a hemodynamically significant LVOT obstruction in 6 patients (9.3%) after valve deployment. The average peak LVOT gradient in these patients was 72 mm Hg (range, 39–100 mm Hg). In a more recently published study of 194 patients undergoing TMVR (107 ViV patients, 50 ViR patients, and 37 valve-in-MAC patients) the investigators encountered LVOT obstruction in 26 (13.4%), with a significantly higher rate in the valve-in-MAC group compared with the ViR and ViV groups (54.1% vs 8.0% vs 1.9%; $P<.001$).[22] Of note, no differences in the occurrence of LVOT obstruction were found between the different types of transcatheter heart valves, sizes of transcatheter heart valves, or access site used. In the evolving era of TMVR, larger scale study of consecutive patients will be needed to define the actual prevalence of LVOT obstruction following implantation of different transcatheter heart valves.

Outcomes of Left Ventricular Outflow Tract Obstruction Following Transcatheter Mitral Valve Replacement

Limited data have been accumulated to date regarding the clinical outcomes of LVOT obstruction following TMVR. Guerrero and colleagues[19] reported the outcomes of 64 patients from 32 centers who underwent TMVR with compassionate use of balloon-expandable valves. The mean patient age was 73 ± 13 years, 66% were women, and the mean Society of Thoracic Surgeons predicted operative mortality score was 14.4 ± 9.5%. Access was transatrial in 15.6%, transapical in 43.8%, and transseptal in 40.6%. Thirty-day all-cause mortality was 29.7%; 84% of the survivors with follow-up data available were in NYHA functional class I–II at 30 days (n = 25). Among the 6 patients (9.3%) who had LVOT obstruction with hemodynamically significant compromise, mortality was high (83%): 1 patient died during the procedure; 1 was stabilized medically but died of pneumonia 9 days later; 1 was converted to open surgery for valve retrieval and died hours later; 1 was treated with simultaneous kissing aortic and mitral balloon valvuloplasty with significant improvement in LVOT gradient but died 48 hours later due to multiorgan failure; 1 was treated with emergent percutaneous alcohol septal ablation with resolution of the gradient and hemodynamic recovery but died 4 days later of complete heart block secondary to the ablation; and 1 patient was treated successfully with emergent alcohol septal ablation and was discharged home. Recently, Yoon and colleagues described the outcomes of TMVR in 194 patients of whom 26 patients (13.4%) developed LVOT obstruction. In their study, patients with LVOT obstruction had significantly higher procedural mortality compared with those without LVOT obstruction (34.6% vs 2.4%; $P<.001$).

IMAGING FOR TRANSCATHETER MITRAL VALVE REPLACEMENT—PREDICTING LEFT VENTRICULAR OUTFLOW TRACT OBSTRUCTION AND PERIPROCEDURAL IMAGING

Imaging assessment of the mitral valve anatomy is crucial before TMVR procedures and the essentials of imaging include computed tomography (CT) and transesophageal echo, summarized in Table 2.

Computed Tomography

CT is the main imaging modality for pre-TMVR device sizing and assessment of potential procedural obstacles. The mitral annulus has a nonplanar, saddle-shaped configuration with the posterior peak formed by the insertion of the PML and the anterior/aortic peak being continuous with the aortic annulus. This complex nonplanar 3-dimensional (3D) circumference can be delineated on CT by segmental tracing of the mitral annulus during stepwise rotation around the left ventricular long axis.[23] Noticeably, the anterior projection of the saddle-shaped annulus protrudes into the LVOT trajectory. Implantation of a transcatheter heart valve in the anterior projection axis would be thus likely to cause LVOT obstruction.[23] Accordingly, it has thus been proposed that the mitral annulus should rather be addressed in pre-TMVR imaging as a D-shaped structure, and[24] this can be achieved by linear

Table 2 Imaging essentials for TMVR and evaluation of LVOT obstruction	
Echocardiography	**Computed Tomography**
Transthoracic echo (TTE) • Evaluation of LV size and function • Assessment of wall thickness and septal hypertrophy and baseline LVOT gradient • Evaluation of anterior and posterior mitral leaflets and redundancy • Presence of preexisting SAM or chordal SAM Transesophageal Echo (TEE) • Assessment of dynamic LVOT obstruction during TMVR procedure • Confirm valve positioning and function	• Assessment of aortomitral angle • Evaluation of mitral annular calcification • Measurement of neo-LVOT • Device selection using specific models to predict neo-LVOT measurements • May be useful for generation of 3D printed models for procedure planning

tracing of the distance between by medial and lateral fibrous trigones, excluding the anterior aortomitral continuity.[24] The "neo-LVOT" and its trajectory can be then evaluated readily using virtual simulation of transcatheter heart valve implantation. Eventually, the newly formed annular D shape has a smaller circumference and is considerably more planar than the native saddle shape. This allows the design of an S curve of orthogonal fluoroscopic views that may assist device implantation.[25]

Wang and colleagues[18] demonstrated the validity of preprocedural computer-aided virtual simulation models for prediction of LVOT obstruction following TMVR in 38 patients with degenerative surgical mitral ring, bioprosthesis, or severe native MAC. The neo-LVOT area was efficiently predicted ($R^2 = 0.8169$, $P<.0001$) by pre-TMVR LVOT modeling, on validation with post-TMVR CT measurements.[18] In their study, a predicted neo-LVOT surface area of less than or equal to 189.4 mm^2 was found to have 100% sensitivity and 96.8% specificity for prediction of TMVR-associated LVOT obstruction.[18] Integration of computer-assisted design and generation of 3D printing of heart models has been also suggested for accurate ex vivo bench testing of mitral transcatheter heart valves in patient-specific anatomy.[15,26] Three-dimensional models can be physically generated with putative transcatheter heart valves deployed in different left ventricular landing zones/depth of implantation within the patient's mitral annulus, ring, or bioprosthesis. The post-TMVR neo-LVOT area can be then assessed for the proposed transcatheter heart valve by various depths of left ventricular deployment and angulations of the transcatheter heart valve delivery system.[26] Ultimately, computer-assisted tomography and printing allow personalized estimation of patient-specific 3D anatomy, overcoming the main limitation of traditional 2D imaging planes.

Transesophageal Echocardiography

The compound structure and function of the native mitral valve mandates a thorough preprocedural imaging assessment.[27] Transesophageal echocardiography (TEE) is well established in assessment of dynamic LVOT obstruction in hypertrophic cardiomyopathy and in predicting SAM following mitral valve surgery.[28] Recent pilot studies have shown that 3D-TEE might be effective in the prediction of LVOT obstruction in patients undergoing transcatheter ViV intervention, by assessment of the spatial relationship between the existing mitral bioprosthetic struts and the intraventricular septum[29] as well as the intraprocedural changes in the aortomitral angle.[30]

LVOT obstruction can be evaluated and diagnosed by TEE during the TMVR procedure. TEE may demonstrate a narrowed LVOT with displacement of the AML toward the LVOT that can be either fixed or dynamic. In the setting of ViV, the stent struts of the transcatheter heart valve are often detectable on TEE within the LVOT.[30] Doppler echocardiography is also useful to detect an elevated peak gradient across the LVOT. Invasive hemodynamic monitoring during the TMVR procedure is essential to recognize the hemodynamic effects of LVOT obstruction, assess the level of obstruction within the outflow tract, and monitor the response to treatment.

THERAPEUTIC OPTIONS FOR LEFT VENTRICULAR OUTFLOW TRACT OBSTRUCTION POST-TRANSCATHETER MITRAL VALVE REPLACEMENT

The first-line therapy for LVOT obstruction in hemodynamically stable patients is medical management (Table 3). In many cases, small

Table 3
Therapeutic options for LVOT obstruction following TMVR procedures

Medical Management	• Volume loading • Vasopressors • Beta-blockers in the setting of tachyarrhythmias
Alcohol Septal Ablation	• May be considered in the setting of acute obstruction although limited evidence • Some advocate performing procedure before TMVR in high-risk cases; however there is limited evidence
LAMPOON (Laceration of the AML to Prevent LVOT ObstructioN)	• Laceration of the anterior mitral leaflet performed before TMVR to limit obstruction caused by SAM • Being studied in a clinical trial; limited evidence to date
Perfusion Balloon Inflation in LVOT	• Perfusion balloon inflated in the LVOT to maintain patency during TMVR deployment preventing protrusion of TMVR into LVOT • Case report only; limited evidence

ventricular dimensions and hypercontractility contribute to LVOT obstruction and therefore ensuring adequate volume status with intravenous volume loading is of key importance. Inotropes should be used carefully with the understanding that inotropes and vasodilators may exacerbate dynamic obstruction, as in the case of hypertrophic obstructive cardiomyopathy. The use of beta-blockers should be considered in the setting of tachycardia as well as vasoconstricting agents to increase afterload.[31] In the current era of new pharmacologic agents for the treatment of heart failure, such as Entresto (sacubitril/valsartan), which is a powerful vasodilator,[32] consideration should be given to suspending these medications, before the intervention and until other contributing factors, such as dehydration or tachycardia, have resolved.

In the setting of hemodynamic compromise there have been several reports of urgent percutaneous alcohol septal ablation performed to reduce LVOT obstruction.[16,33] Alcohol septal ablation is a transcatheter therapy used for the treatment of LVOT obstruction in patients with hypertrophic cardiomyopathy.[34] Alcohol is selectively injected into septal branches of the left anterior descending artery that perfuse the obstructive segment of the interventricular septum, resulting in a confined myocardial infarction. This results in a reduction of the LVOT gradient that shows comparable efficacy to that of surgical septal myectomy in terms of mortality, functional status, ventricular arrhythmia, reinterventions, and postprocedure mitral regurgitation.[35] Complications of alcohol septal ablation include, however, permanent atrioventricular block in approximately 10% of patients.[35] Successful use of alcohol septal ablation was previously described to treat LVOT obstruction following mitral valve annuloplasty.[16] Later, individual case reports have demonstrated the hemodynamic benefits of alcohol septal ablation for the treatment of acute LVOT obstruction following transcatheter mitral valve-in-MAC procedures.[33,36] Likewise, a recent small series of patients treated with alcohol septal ablation following valve-in-MAC also demonstrated acute postprocedural amelioration in LVOT gradients (Fig. 2).[37] Early results of incorporation of preemptive alcohol septal ablation before TMVR in patients stratified as high risk for LVOT obstruction postprocedure have shown this technique to be feasible in the hands of centers with experience with alcohol septal ablation and treatment of hypertrophic cardiomyopathy. Alcohol septal ablation is a relatively simple procedure, although it has

been associated with different degrees of atrioventricular block, need for permanent pacemaker implantation, and malignant arrhythmias.[34] Therefore, thoughtful consideration should be given before recommending this therapy routinely for patients with TMVR.

Alternative approaches to the management of LVOT obstruction focus on primary prevention before prosthesis implantation to circumvent later hemodynamic compromise. Two different methods have been proposed for prevention of LVOT obstruction. The first involves laceration of the AML before mitral valve implantation[38] and the other aims to preserve LVOT patency by concomitant balloon inflation during transcatheter heart valve deployment.

SAM has been identified as a causative factor in both fixed and dynamic LVOT obstruction. As described by Greenbaum and colleagues, an elongated AML may interfere directly with the functioning of an implanted transcatheter valve in the mitral position by prolapsing through the valve or may affect closure of the leaflets of the bioprosthetic valve. Additional factors such as volume depletion may worsen a dynamic obstruction provoked by the AML protrusion into the LVOT. A new percutaneous approach has been studied in animals to establish proof of concept and involves the intentional laceration of the A2 segment of the mitral valve using a coronary wire and radiofrequency ablation.[39] This technique, named LAMPOON, or laceration of the AML to prevent LVOT obstruction procedure, requires retrograde access to the left

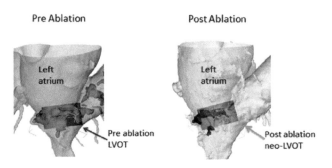

Pre Ablation   Post Ablation

Left atrium   Left atrium

Pre ablation LVOT   Post ablation neo-LVOT

Fig. 2. CT analysis of neo-LVOT pre- and postalcohol septal ablation.

	Position (LV/LA)	Predicted Neo-LVOT surface area (mm2)
Pre- Ablation	80/20	24
Post alcohol septal ablation	80/20	223

atrium via the aortic valve and placement of 2 coronary guiding catheters, one in the LVOT adjacent to the aortomitral curtain and the other in the left atrium. A coronary guidewire is then advanced through an insulated polymer jacket via the LVOT catheter and electrified to perforate the anterior mitral leaflet and is then snared by the catheter to form a loop in the left atrium. This loop is then energized and withdrawn, lacerating the A2 segment of the AML. The procedure successfully lacerated the anterior leaflet in the animals studied without evidence of chordal disruption.[39]

The LAMPOON procedure has been also tested to prevent LVOT obstruction in 5 patients with mitral valve disease and prohibitive surgical risk before transcatheter mitral valve intervention.[38] Preprocedural imaging is crucial in planning for LAMPOON. To ensure higher likelihood of success in perforating the leaflet scallop of entrance followed by tear, the anterior mitral leaflet must not be overly calcified. However, despite LAMPOON, Khan and colleagues[40] have demonstrated that there is no true curative prevention for LVOT obstruction in transcatheter valve implantation. The LAMPOON procedure is able to be performed at the time of TMVR but will only be able to increase the predicted neo-LVOT to the level of the skirt of the transcatheter heart valve being implanted. If the predicted skirt neo-LVOT is less than 150 mm^2, there still exists a profound risk of iatrogenic LVOT obstruction. The LAMPOON procedure will be studied further in an early feasibility study funded by the NHLBI (Intentional Laceration of the Anterior Mitral Leaflet to Prevent Left Ventricular Outflow Tract Obstruction During Transcatheter Mitral Valve Implantation, ClinicalTrials.gov Identifier, NCT03015194). A total of 60 patients will be enrolled. Key inclusion criteria include severe symptomatic native mitral valve failure after mitral annuloplasty repair or related to MAC, extremely high or prohibitive risk for surgical mitral valve replacement and indication for TMVR, high or prohibitive risk of LVOT obstruction (predicted neo-LVOT <200 mm^2), or transcatheter heart valve dysfunction due to long/redundant AML, as determined by the multidisciplinary institutional heart team. The primary outcome is technical success at 30 days.

Herrmann and colleagues[41] have recently described the use of a perfusion balloon placed in the LVOT to prevent LVOT obstruction in a case report. The perfusion balloon was advanced retrogradely into the LVOT and inflated under rapid pacing before transcatheter heart valve deployment in the mitral position. The perfusion balloon maintained the patency of the LVOT and permitted outflow while positioning and deploying the prosthetic device. In addition, simultaneous inflation with the mitral valve prosthesis prevented protrusion and overflaring of the mitral prosthesis toward the LVOT. According to the investigators, no significant LVOT obstruction was observed postintervention in this case.[41] This approach has been used in similar cases with a standard valvuloplasty balloon, using a kissing balloon inflation to maintain LVOT patency, identify the landing zone, and orient the transcatheter valve.[42] The long-term implications of such a technique are as yet unknown and require further experience.

LONG-TERM IMPLICATIONS OF LEFT VENTRICULAR OUTFLOW TRACT OBSTRUCTION POST-TRANSCATHETER MITRAL VALVE REPLACEMENT

The long-term outcomes of patients with LVOT obstruction post-TMVR still remain to be clarified. Data gathered from surgical valve repair/replacement complicated by LVOT obstruction have roughly identified 2 main groups of patient: those who can be managed with medical therapy, namely beta-blockade and prevention of hypovolemia, and those requiring further mechanical intervention to resolve obstruction.[43,44] Early experience from transcatheter mitral valve therapies, although scarce, have also showed success with medical therapy,[45] but requirement for repeat interventions in some cases.[46] One of the earliest case series of surgical patients with LVOT obstruction postmitral annuloplasty observed 12 patients postmitral valve repair.[47] In 5 patients, surgical reintervention was required immediately postrepair. In the remaining 7 patients, no further intervention was necessary at 27 months, and there was no evidence of secondary left ventricular hypertrophy on follow-up despite persistent LVOT obstruction. The largest published surgical case series followed the outcomes of 174 patients postmitral valve repair with persistent SAM.[31] In this cohort of patients treated between 1993 and 2002 at the Mayo Clinic, 174 out of 2076 mitral repair patients had evidence of SAM intraoperatively. Of these patients, 20% (n = 34) also had evidence of LVOT obstruction. In most of the cases, SAM resolved before hospital discharge; however, one patient with LVOT obstruction did require surgical removal of the annuloplasty band. Late follow-up (median 4.7 years) was available in 139 patients, amongst whom 4 had

LVOT obstruction, yet no further intervention was required at follow-up.

Insights regarding the long-term impact of LVOT obstruction may be deduced also from the clinical experience with hypertrophic cardiomyopathy, notwithstanding the noticeable disparities between these 2 entities. The 2014 European Society of Cardiology Guidelines for Hypertrophic Cardiomyopathy reiterate the definition of LVOT obstruction as a gradient greater than or equal to 30 mm Hg, while setting the threshold for intervention at greater than or equal to 50 mm Hg.[48] These guidelines endorse general measures such as avoidance of dehydration and medical therapy that may worsen LVOT obstruction. The mainstay of medical therapy is nonvasodilating beta-blockers. Noticeably, there are no data to support treatment of LVOT obstruction in asymptomatic patients. Early studies of patients with hypertrophic cardiomyopathy had identified LVOT obstruction as a risk factor for sudden death in this population at a threshold of 30 mm Hg, yet the likelihood of death did not increase further in those with LVOT gradients above 30 mm Hg.[49] Further work, however, has suggested an increased mortality risk associated with increased LVOT gradient; however, in asymptomatic patients, all-cause mortality was low despite LVOT obstruction, implying that intervention may be unwarranted in the absence of symptoms.[50] LVOT obstruction is a recognized risk factor for sudden death in patients with hypertrophic cardiomyopathy and must be part of risk stratification in these patients.[51] Of note, it is still uncertain whether interventions to decrease LVOT obstruction ameliorate the risks of sudden death in patients with hypertrophic cardiomyopathy. For patients without hypertrophic cardiomyopathy but iatrogenic LVOT obstruction, the risks are even less clear and remain to be elucidated.

SUMMARY

LVOT obstruction is a well-known phenomenon that may occur after surgical mitral valve repair or replacement. Advancements in patient identification and surgical techniques have successfully addressed this issue in most cases. The risk of LVOT obstruction is a major limitation to the wide adoption of TMVR. The risk of TMVR is greatest in the setting of valve-in-MAC, then valve-in-ring, and least (although not zero) with valve-in-valve. Preprocedural imaging, generally by CT, should focus on modeling the potential neo-LVOT area. Potential mechanical intervention to prevent LVOT obstruction in high-risk cases includes intentional laceration of the anterior mitral leaflet (the LAMPOON procedure) or alcohol septal ablation. Kissing balloon inflation or the use of a perfusion balloon has also been proposed. If LVOT obstruction does occur postprocedure, appropriate medical management includes beta-blockade, hydration, and volume resuscitation. Alcohol septal ablation in the setting of TMVR-induced LVOT obstruction may be therapeutic. However, the threshold at which intervention should be performed in the asymptomatic patient is unknown. Novel transcatheter heart valves technologies that proactively address the anterior mitral leaflet may be advantageous.

REFERENCES

1. Termini BA, Jackson PA, Williams CD. Systolic anterior motion of the mitral valve following annuloplasty. J Vasc Surg 1977;11:55–60.
2. Kreindel MS, Schiavone WA, Lever HM, et al. Systolic anterior motion of the mitral valve after carpentier ring valvuloplasty for mitral valve prolapse. Am J Cardiol 1986;57(6):408–12.
3. Mihaileanu S, Marino JP, Chauvaud S, et al. Left ventricular outflow obstruction after mitral valve repair (Carpentier's technique). Proposed mechanisms of disease. Circulation 1988;78(3 Pt 2):I78–84.
4. Lee KS, Stewart WJ, Lever H, et al. Mechanism of outflow tract obstruction causing failed mitral valve repair: anterior displacement of leaflet coaptation. Circulation 1993;88(5 Pt 2):II24–9.
5. Jebara VA, Mihaileanu S, Acar C, et al. Left ventricular outflow tract obstruction after mitral valve repair. Results of the sliding leaflet technique. Circulation 1993;88(5 Pt 2):II30–4.
6. Maslow AD, Regan MM, Haering JM, et al. Echocardiographic predictors of left ventricular outflow tract obstruction and systolic anterior motion of the mitral valve after mitral valve reconstruction for myxomatous valve disease. J Am Coll Cardiol 1999;34(7):2096–104.
7. Varghese R, Itagaki S, Anyanwu AC, et al. Predicting systolic anterior motion after mitral valve reconstruction: using intraoperative transoesophageal echocardiography to identify those at greatest risk. Eur J Cardiothorac Surg 2014;45(1):132–8.
8. Waggoner AD, Pérez JE, Barzilai B, et al. Left ventricular outflow obstruction resulting from insertion of mitral prostheses leaving the native leaflets intact: adverse clinical outcome in seven patients. Am Heart J 1991;122(2):483–8.
9. Esper MDE, Ferdinand MDFD, Aronson MDS, et al. Prosthetic mitral valve replacement: late complications after native valve preservation. Ann Thorac Surg 1997;63(2):541–3.

10. Rietman GW, van der Maaten JMAA, Douglas YL, et al. Echocardiographic diagnosis of left ventricular outflow tract obstruction after mitral valve replacement with subvalvular preservation. Eur J Cardiothorac Surg 2002;22(5):825–7.

11. Okamoto K, Kiso I, Inoue Y, et al. Left ventricular outflow obstruction after mitral valve replacement preserving native anterior leaflet. Ann Thorac Surg 2006;82(2):735–7.

12. Rosendal C, Hien MD, Bruckner T, et al. Left ventricular outflow tract: intraoperative measurement and changes caused by mitral valve surgery. J Am Soc Echocardiogr 2012;25(2):166–72.

13. Asgar A, Ducharme A, Messas N, et al. Left ventricular outflow tract obstruction following mitral valve replacement: challenges for transcatheter mitral valve therapy. Structural Heart 2018;2(5):372–9.

14. Blanke P, Naoum C, Dvir D, et al. Predicting LVOT obstruction in transcatheter mitral valve implantation: Concept of the Neo-LVOT. JACC Cardiovasc Imaging 2017;10(4):482–5.

15. Wang DD, Eng M, Greenbaum A, et al. Predicting LVOT obstruction after TMVR. JACC Cardiovasc Imaging 2016;9(11):1349.

16. Descoutures F, Himbert D, Maisano F, et al. Transcatheter valve-in-ring implantation after failure of surgical mitral repair. Eur J Cardiothorac Surg 2013;44(1):e8–15.

17. Tang GH-L, Khan MH, Zaid S, et al. changes in aortomitral annular angle after transcatheter aortic valve replacement: implications for transcatheter mitral valve replacement? J Am Coll Cardiol 2018;71(11 Supplement):A1294.

18. Wang DD, Eng MH, Greenbaum AB, et al. Validating a prediction modeling tool for left ventricular outflow tract (LVOT) obstruction after transcatheter mitral valve replacement (TMVR). Catheter Cardiovasc Interv 2018;92(2):379–87.

19. Guerrero M, Urena M, Himbert D, et al. 1-year outcomes of transcatheter mitral valve replacement in patients with severe mitral annular calcification. J Am Coll Cardiol 2018;71(17):1841–53.

20. Bapat V, Pirone F, Kapetanakis S, et al. Factors influencing left ventricular outflow tract obstruction following a mitral valve-in-valve or valve-in-ring procedure, part 1. Catheter Cardiovasc Interv 2015;86(4):747–60.

21. Guler N, Ozkara C, Akyol A. Left ventricular outflow tract obstruction after bioprosthetic mitral valve replacement with posterior mitral leaflet preservation. Tex Heart Inst J 2006;33(3):399–401.

22. Yoon S-H, Bleiziffer S, Latib A, et al. Predictors of left ventricular outflow tract obstruction after transcatheter mitral valve replacement. JACC Cardiovasc Interv 2019;12(2):182–93.

23. Blanke P, Naoum C, Dvir D, et al. Predicting LVOT obstruction in transcatheter mitral valve implantation: concept of the neo-LVOT. JACC Cardiovasc Imaging 2017;10(4):482–5.

24. Blanke P, chavar p, Cheung A, et al. Mitral annular evaluation with CT in the context of transcatheter mitral valve replacement. JACC Cardiovasc Imaging 2015;8:612–5.

25. Pighi M, Theriault-Lauzier P, Piazza N. Multimodality imaging for interventional cardiologists. EuroIntervention 2018;14(AB):AB33–9.

26. Kohli K, Wei ZA, Yoganathan AP, et al. Transcatheter mitral valve planning and the neo-LVOT: utilization of virtual simulation models and 3D printing. Curr Treat Options Cardiovasc Med 2018;20(12):99.

27. Backer OD, Piazza N, Banai S, et al. Percutaneous transcatheter mitral valve replacement. Circ Cardiovasc Interv 2014;7(3):400–9.

28. Cummisford KM, Manning W, Karthik S, et al. 3D TEE and systolic anterior motion in hypertrophic cardiomyopathy. JACC Cardiovasc Imaging 2010; 3(10):1083.

29. Hanson R, Nyman C, Shook DC, et al. Identifying patients at risk for LVOT obstruction in mitral valve-in-valve implantation. JACC Cardiovasc Imaging 2017;10(1):89.

30. Hayashi A, Yoshida J, Yamaguchi S, et al. Echocardiographic assessment of left ventricular outflow tract after transcatheter mitral valve replacement. J Am Coll Cardiol 2018;71(11 Supplement):A1090.

31. Brown ML, Abel MD, Click RL, et al. Systolic anterior motion after mitral valve repair: is surgical intervention necessary? J Thorac Cardiovasc Surg 2007; 133:136–43.

32. Bohm M, Young R, Jhund PS, et al. Systolic blood pressure, cardiovascular outcomes and efficacy and safety of sacubitril/valsartan (LCZ696) in patients with chronic heart failure and reduced ejection fraction: results from PARADIGM-HF. Eur Heart J 2017;38(15):1132–43.

33. Guerrero M, Wang DD, O'Neill W. Percutaneous alcohol septal ablation to acutely reduce left ventricular outflow tract obstruction induced by transcatheter mitral valve replacement. Catheter Cardiovasc Interv 2016;88(6):E191–7.

34. Liebregts M, Vriesendorp PA, ten Berg JM. Alcohol septal ablation for obstructive hypertrophic cardiomyopathy. J Am Coll Cardiol 2017;70(4):481.

35. Agarwal S, Tuzcu EM, Desai MY, et al. Updated meta-analysis of septal alcohol ablation versus myectomy for hypertrophic cardiomyopathy. J Am Coll Cardiol 2010;55(8):823.

36. Deharo P, Urena M, Himbert D, et al. Bail-out alcohol septal ablation for left ventricular outflow tract obstruction after transcatheter mitral valve replacement. JACC Cardiovasc Interv 2016;9(8):e73–6.

37. Guerrero M, Wang DD, Himbert D, et al. Short-term results of alcohol septal ablation as a bail-out strategy to treat severe left ventricular outflow

tract obstruction after transcatheter mitral valve replacement in patients with severe mitral annular calcification. Catheter Cardiovasc Interv 2017; 90(7):1220–6.

38. Babaliaros VC, Greenbaum AB, Khan JM, et al. Intentional percutaneous laceration of the anterior mitral leaflet to prevent outflow obstruction during transcatheter mitral valve replacement: first-in-human experience. JACC Cardiovasc Interv 2017; 10(8):798–809.

39. Khan JM, Rogers T, Schenke WH, et al. Intentional laceration of the anterior mitral valve leaflet to prevent left ventricular outflow tract obstruction during transcatheter mitral valve replacement: pre-clinical findings. JACC Cardiovasc Interv 2016;9(17):1835–43.

40. Khan JM, Rogers T, Babaliaros VC, et al. Predicting left ventricular outflow tract obstruction despite anterior mitral leaflet resection: the "Skirt NeoLVOT". JACC Cardiovasc Imaging 2018;11(9):1356–9.

41. Herrmann HC, Szeto WY, Litt H, et al. Novel use of perfusion balloon inflation to avoid outflow tract obstruction during transcatheter mitral valve-in-valve replacement. Catheter Cardiovasc Interv 2018;92(3):601–6.

42. Rahhab Z, Ren B, de Jaegere PPT, et al. Kissing balloon technique to secure the neo-left ventricular outflow tract in transcatheter mitral valve implantation. Eur Heart J 2018;39(23):2220.

43. Watt J, Hogg KJ, Danton M. Resolution of dynamic left ventricular outflow tract obstruction caused by retained native leaflets following mitral valve replacement using medical treatment. Heart 2006; 92(9):1318.

44. Lee J, Tey KR, Mizyed A, et al. Mitral valve replacement complicated by iatrogenic left ventricular outflow obstruction and paravalvular leak: case report and review of literature. BMC Cardiovasc Disord 2015;15:119.

45. Alsidawi S, Eleid MF, Rihal CS, et al. Significant LVOT obstruction after mitral valve in ring procedure. Eur Heart J Cardiovasc Imaging 2015;16(12): 1389.

46. Said SM, Pislaru S, Kotkar KD, et al. Left ventricular outflow tract obstruction after transcatheter mitral valve-in-ring implantation: a word of caution. Ann Thorac Surg 2016;102(6):e495–7.

47. Schiavone W, Cosgrove M, Lever H, et al. Long-term follow-up of patients with left ventricular outflow tract obstruction after Carpentier ring mitral valvuloplasty. Circulation 1988;78(3 Pt 2): 160–5.

48. Authors/Task Force members, Elliott PM, Anastasakis A, Borger MA, et al. 2014 ESC guidelines on diagnosis and management of hypertrophic cardiomyopathyThe task force for the diagnosis and management of hypertrophic cardiomyopathy of the European Society of Cardiology (ESC). Eur Heart J 2014;35(39):2733–79.

49. Maron MS, Olivotto I, Betocchi S, et al. Effect of left ventricular outflow tract obstruction on clinical outcome in hypertrophic cardiomyopathy. N Engl J Med 2003;348(4):295–303.

50. Elliott PM, Gimeno JR, Tomé MT, et al. Left ventricular outflow tract obstruction and sudden death risk in patients with hypertrophic cardiomyopathy. Eur Heart J 2006;27(16):1933–41.

51. Obadia JF, Messika-Zeitoun D, Leurent G, et al. Percutaneous repair or medical treatment for secondary mitral regurgitation. N Engl J Med 2018; 379(24):2297–306.

Prevention and Treatment of Left Ventricular Outflow Tract Obstruction After Transcatheter Mitral Valve Replacement

John Lisko, MD, MPH[a], Norihiko Kamioka, MD[a],
Patrick Gleason, MD[a], Isida Byku, MD[a],
Lucia Alvarez, MD[a], Jaffar M. Khan, BM, BCh[b],
Toby Rogers, PhD, BM, BCh[c], Robert Lederman, MD[c],
Adam Greenbaum, MD[a], Vasilis Babaliaros, MD[a],*

KEYWORDS

- Transcatheter mitral valve replacement • LVOT Obstruction • LAMPOON • Neo-LVOT
- Skirt NEO-LVOT

KEY POINTS

- Transcatheter mitral valve replacement is a promising strategy for patients with severe mitral valve disease and no surgical options.
- Left ventricular outflow tract obstruction is a life-threatening complication of transcatheter mitral valve replacement. There are currently no commercially available devices to prevent left ventricular outflow tract obstruction.
- Multiple techniques to prevent left ventricular outflow tract obstruction have been developed by modifying current devices.
- The LAMPOON technique is a promising strategy using electrosurgical techniques to reduce the risk of left ventricular outflow tract obstruction.

CASE

An 84-year-old Caucasian woman with a past medical history significant for coronary artery disease status post 3 vessel coronary artery bypass grafting, mitral valve repair with a mitral ring, chronic kidney disease stage IV, chronic obstructive pulmonary disease not on home oxygen, and insulin-dependent diabetes presents to the Structural Heart and Valve clinic with a chief complaint of worsening shortness of breath. An echocardiogram reveals severe mitral regurgitation (regurgitant fraction, 45%, effective regurgitant orifice [ERO], 0.46 mm^2), mean gradient, 3 mm Hg). Her Society of Thoracic Surgery predicted operative mortality risk score calculates to 9.4%. The heart team deems her to be a candidate for a valve-in-ring transcatheter

---

Disclosure Statement: Dr V. Babaliaros is a consultant for both Edwards and Abbott. Dr A. Greenbaum is a consultant for both Edwards and Abbott. Dr T. Rogers is a consultant/proctor for Edwards Lifesciences and Medtronic.
[a] Division of Cardiology, Emory University, 1639 Pierce Drive, Atlanta, GA 30322, USA; [b] Division of Cardiology, Washington Hospital Center, 110 Irving Street, Northwest, Washington, DC 20010, USA; [c] Cardiovascular Branch, Division of Intramural Research, National Heart Lung and Blood Institute, National Institutes of Health, Building 10, Room 2c713, MSC 1538, Bethesda, MD 20892-1538, USA
* Corresponding author. Structural Heart and Valve Center, Emory University Midtown Hospital, 550 Peachtree St NE, Atlanta, GA 30308.
E-mail address: vbabali@emory.edu

mitral valve replacement (TMVR); however, her preprocedural planning computed tomography (CT) scan demonstrates a thickened interventricular septum and concern for left ventricular outflow tract (LVOT) obstruction.

INTRODUCTION

TMVR is becoming a viable option for patients with severe mitral valve disease and no surgical options.[1] LVOT obstruction is a known complication of TMVR that portends a poor prognosis.[2] This review discusses the current state of TMVR and reviews strategies to prevent LVOT obstruction, with an emphasis on Heart Team decision-making and promising prophylactic, electrosurgical techniques to modify the mitral valve leaflets before valve implantation.

TRANSCATHETER MITRAL VALVE REPLACEMENT

The advent of transcatheter aortic valve replacement (TAVR) began a revolution in the treatment of valvular heart disease. Over the past decade, skills and technology previously used in the aortic space have been modified for the treatment of mitral valve disorders. Transcatheter mitral valve replacement (TMVR) has become a possible treatment for patients with mitral stenosis or regurgitation and no surgical options.

Currently, there are no commercially dedicated TMVR systems.[1] Available options are limited to clinical trials or the off-label use of balloon expandable aortic valves modified for the mitral position. All current transcatheter mitral valves available under research protocols require transapical placement, whereas the Edwards Sapien Valve (Edwards Life Science, Irvine, CA) (Fig. 1) can be delivered either transapically or transseptally. Given the risk profile of this patient cohort and that most devices are either first-generation or off-label, postprocedure mortality remains high.[2]

TMVR is feasible for valve-in-surgical valve (V-i-V) procedures,[3] valve in prior surgically placed mitral rings, and valve-in-mitral annular calcification (MAC).[4] Of the 3 interventions, V-i-V is the least technically challenging, given the support of the prior valve frame and the known inner diameter of the prosthetic valve, which is useful for sizing purposes. The annuloplasty ring during mitral valve-in-ring therapy also provides an anchor for TMVR deployment but procedural outcomes are limited by potential ring dehiscence and limitations in valve deployment. TMVR in MAC is the most technically challenging replacement to perform and requires a circumferential ring of calcium. Valve deployment may be limited by the uneven nature of MAC and leads to paravalvular leak.[5]

As TMVR is a relatively new approach to the treatment of mitral valve disease, no large-scale randomized trials have been completed to date. In a large multicenter registry of valve-in-MAC, initial success was reported in 76.6% of cases and 46.3% of patients were alive at 1 year. Notably, 11.2% of patients experienced LVOT obstruction with hemodynamic compromise. Of these 13 patients, only 2 were alive at 1-year follow-up. When outcomes were stratified by operator experience, there was no statistically difference in the rate of LVOT between early and late experience.[2]

LEFT VENTRICULAR OUTFLOW TRACT OBSTRUCTION

LVOT obstruction from permanent displacement of the anterior mitral valve leaflet is more common in valve-in-ring and valve-in-MAC procedures. In addition, approximately 50% of patients are excluded from clinical trials given the risk of LVOT obstruction. Given the significant nature of this problem, much work has focused on the prediction, prevention, and treatment of LVOT obstruction.[6]

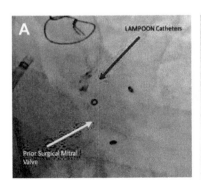
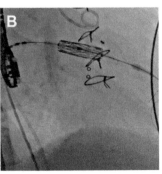

Fig. 1. (A, B) S3 valve positioning for V-i-V TMVR post LAMPOON. (*Courtesy of* Edwards Lifesciences, Irvine, CA.)

Defining the Left Ventricular Outflow Tract

The anterior mitral valve leaflet (AML) physically separates the inflow and outflow zones of the left ventricle. Before TMVR, the AML moves into the LVOT during diastole and retracts out of the LVOT during systole. During TMVR, valve struts can be either circumferentially covered or the anterior mitral leaflet will be placed in a permanently "open" position creating a neo-LVOT.[7] In certain at-risk patients, the AML may encroach into the LVOT, causing obstruction and a functional subaortic stenosis. Given the significant mortality associated with LVOT obstruction, detailed preprocedural CT assessment is essential to comprehensively evaluate risk. Threatened LVOT obstruction is an exclusion criteria for approximately 50% of patients in contemporary clinical trials.[6]

Preprocedural 3-dimensional CT allows for the accurate modeling of cardiac anatomy and deployment of a virtual transcatheter heart valve. The mitral valve plane is defined as the basalmost insertion point of the mitral valve leaflets. In most cases, using a gated cardiac CT, this plane should be measured at 40% of the cardiac cycle to determine the narrowest possible neo-LVOT. Using the double-oblique method, the plane can be measured in both sagittal and coronal cross section. Using these dimensions, a valve size can be determined and a virtual valve can be placed.[8] The valve is typically placed 80% ventricular and 20% atrial; however, it should be modeled at various positions in the event of valve migration during deployment.[9] LVOT surface areas can be obtained after virtual valve placement, and a neo-LVOT area can be determined. Retrospective analysis of 38 patients undergoing TMVR determined that a neo-LVOT area ≤189 mm² portended a higher risk of LVOT obstruction[10] (Fig. 2).

Aorto-mitral angulation, left ventricular (LV) size, and interventricular septal size are also essential for a comprehensive assessment of LVOT obstruction risk. In general, as the angle between the aortic and mitral angle approaches 90° and LV size decreases, the risk of LVOT obstruction increases.[11]

Prevention of Left Ventricular Outflow Tract Obstruction

Surgical splitting of the anterior mitral valve leaflet

David's[12] technique allows for splitting of the anterior mitral leaflet during open cardiac surgery. In patients at risk of LVOT obstruction, a hybrid approach to valve replacement that involves surgical laceration followed by TMVR is feasible, especially given advancements in minimally invasive and robotic mitral surgery. However, the cardiac risk profile of most patients undergoing TMVR precludes them from any form of cardiac surgery. Because of this, the remainder of this review will focus on solely catheter-based solutions to LVOT obstruction.

Alcohol septal ablation

Alcohol septal ablation, a noninvasive technique to reduce septal musculature, is used as a therapeutic strategy in patients with hypertrophic obstructive cardiomyopathy. Case reports have also described alcohol septal ablation to reduce LVOT obstruction post-TMVR.[13,14] However, this procedure is limited in patients with a relatively thin interventricular septum. The septal pathway of the His-Purkinje system also increases the risk of postablation complete heart block necessitating permeant pacemaker implantation.

To date, the only systematic study of patients who have undergone this technique as a "bailout" strategy is limited to a report of 6 patients

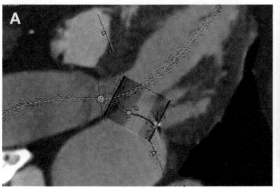
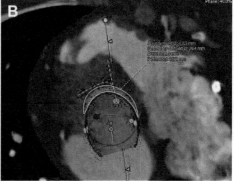

Fig. 2. CT assessment for LVOT obstruction. Detailed preprocedure CT analysis allows for assessment of LVOT obstruction risk. Note, measurements are performed in the 40% phase of the cardiac cycle with the valve placed so that 20% is atrial and 80% ventricular (A). In this patient, the neo-LVOT area of 118.9 mm² (B) predicts a high risk of LVOT obstruction after TMVR.

treated at 6 different centers. In this cohort, 5 patients had immediate reduction in LVOT gradient and 4 were alive at 30 days.[15] There have been no prospective studies of alcohol septal ablation before TMVR. Applying this strategy to selected patients may prove to be a viable alternative to preemptive splitting of the anterior leaflet; however, the need for myocardial remodeling necessitates approximately a 6-week waiting period. Also, there is a mortality risk from this procedure as a stand-alone prevention strategy.

Radiofrequency ablation

Alcohol septal ablation is not a viable strategy to prevent LVOT obstruction in patients with an anatomically unsuitable septal perforator or a thin interventricular septum. Although still investigational in nature, radiofrequency ablation of the interventricular septum may be a viable strategy for these patients. This procedure does not require preprocedure CT and can be guided by transesophageal echocardiography (TEE). Using techniques originally designed for arrhythmia ablation, radiofrequency catheters can be placed near the predicted area of LVOT obstruction (Fig. 3). After ablating the myocardium, it becomes dyskinetic or akinetic, thereby creating a larger neo-LVOT. This procedure has been used twice in our institution and its long-term outcomes are unknown. The limitations of this technique relegate its use to a compassionate basis.

Intentional percutaneous laceration of the anterior mitral leaflet to prevent outflow obstruction

The LAMPOON (Intentional Percutaneous Laceration of the Anterior Mitral Leaflet to Prevent Outflow Obstruction) technique was developed to mitigate the risk of LVOT obstruction before TMVR with a Sapien valve in the mitral position. LAMPOON uses transcatheter electrosurgery to mimic David's[12] surgical anterior resection with chordal sparing (Fig. 4). As there are no commercially available catheters for LAMPOON, the technique was developed using modified commercially available devices.[7]

In the first step of the procedure, two 6-French coronary guiding catheters are advanced across the aortic valve. One catheter is positioned in the LVOT at the base of the A2 scallop and the other catheter is placed retrograde into the left atrium. Electrosurgical crossing is achieved by modification of techniques used for transcaval TAVR access. First an insulating polymer jacket wire converter (Piggyback, Teleflex, Morrisville, NC) is placed inside of the LVOT catheter. For electrosurgical crossing, a 0.014-inch by 300 cm guide wire is placed through this jacket and electrified at 50W (pure cut). Once the wire passes through the base of the A2 scallop it is captured by a snare placed in the left atrium and externalized (Fig. 5).

Once externalized, a segment of the guidewire is denuded and kinked. By kinking the wire, energy can be focused on the inner curvature, which is positioned in the anterior mitral leaflet. Again, the guidewire is electrified and pulled back to fully split the anterior mitral leaflet. During this electrification, dextrose is injected to avoid the dispersion of charge from the blood's iron content.[6]

The first-in-human experience was systematically studied in 5 patients with prohibitive risk of LVOT obstruction before TMVR. Of these 5 patients, 3 had a prior mitral ring, 1 had a prior

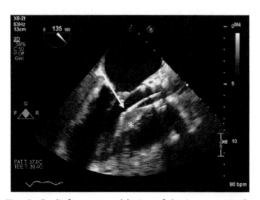

Fig. 3. Radiofrequency ablation of the interventricular septum using TEE guidance. Radiofrequency ablation catheters (*arrow*) can be used to ablate the interventricular septum (*star*) when there are no anatomically suitable septal perforators for alcohol septal ablation.

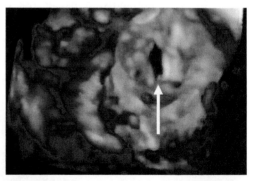

Fig. 4. Anterior mitral leaflet post LAMPOON. Three-dimensional TEE of a lacerated AML. This technique decreases the risk of LVOT obstruction by allowing for blood flow through open transcatheter heart valve cells that otherwise would be covered by the anterior mitral leaflet. The arrow is pointing to the "split" anterior mitral valve leaflet post LAMPOON.

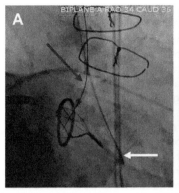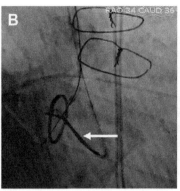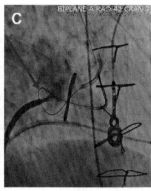

Fig. 5. LAMPOON technique. The LAMPOON technique was developed using modifications of commercially available devices. (*A*) A snare is placed in the left atrium (*white arrow*) and a guidewire is placed in the LVOT catheter (*red arrow*). The guidewire is electrified, passed through the base of the A2 scallop, and snared in the left atrium (*B*). The wire is then externalized, kinked, and positioned at the base of the anterior leaflet. Once electrified, the wire can traverse and lacerate the anterior leaflet decreasing obstruction risk post-TMVR (*C*).

mitral band, and 1 had MAC. Results of this original work were promising with 80% survival at 30 days and no significant paravalvular leak, major bleeding, or vascular complications. No patients in the original study had a critical LVOT gradient after TMVR and there were no impediments to function of the transcatheter heart valve.[6]

Following the results of this experience, an early feasibility trial was conducted to study LAMPOON in a larger population. This multicenter center included 30 subjects who were ineligible for isolated TMVR and were poor candidates for other clinical trials. This cohort had a risk of severe LVOT obstruction from either a skirt neo-LVOT of less than 150 mm² or a long redundant anterior mitral leaflet. In this cohort, 100% of patients had successful traversal of the AML, laceration of the AML, and TMVR implantation. In-hospital survival in this study was 93%, which is significantly higher than reported in other clinical trials. Seventy percent of patients met criteria for technical success and did not require emergency surgery, bail-out alcohol septal ablation, unplanned paravalvular leak device closure, or need for a second valve, consistent with the limitations of using an off-label Sapien valve in the mitral position.

Four patients in the LAMPOON IDE had an LVOT gradient greater than 30 mm Hg after TMVR deployment. Review of postprocedure CT images suggested that insufficient laceration (tip laceration, n = 1) and the valve skirt of the S3 (n = 3) can create LVOT obstruction (the concept of a "skirt" neo-LVOT measurement). Patients with a "skirt neo-LVOT" of less than 150 mm²[16] will likely require adjunctive procedures, such as alcohol or radiofrequency septal ablation (Fig. 6). Although further validation is still needed, measuring skirt neo-LVOT appears

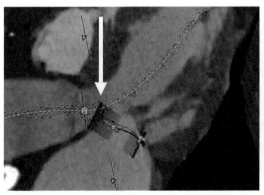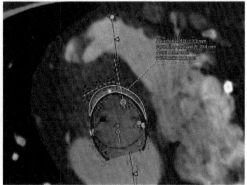

Fig. 6. CT assessment for "skirt" obstruction. After TMVR, the valve skirt can protrude in the LVOT. As this is a fixed structure, LVOT obstruction can occur despite successful laceration of the anterior mitral leaflet. After assessment of the neo-LVOT, the "skirt" neo-LVOT should be modeled by simulating a virtual valve skirt (*arrow*) and measuring the predicted area (*asterisk*). Patients with a "skirt" neo-LVOT of less than 150 mm² will often require an adjunctive procedure to decrease the risk of obstruction.

to be a necessary additional measurement before TMVR.

Our center has also applied the LAMPOON technique to patients with bioprosthetic mitral valve replacement before transcatheter valve-in-valve procedures. Using standard LAMPOON techniques, the anterior leaflet of the bioprosthetic valve was lacerated and the Sapien valve was deployed without significant LVOT obstruction. Although the technique has not been systematically studied in this population, it appears that LAMPOON is a viable strategy for patients with prior bioprosthetic valves who are at high risk of LVOT obstruction.

In addition to the standard assessments of the neo-LVOT, anterior mitral leaflet length (>24 mm) should be carefully assessed before TMVR. A case series by Greenbaum and colleagues[17] describes 3 patients with long or redundant anterior mitral leaflets undergoing TMVR. In this cohort, the anterior mitral leaflet interfered with transcatheter heart valve function by either prolapsing through the valve, preventing valve pressurization, or causing a dynamic LVOT obstruction. LAMPOON is a viable preventive strategy preventing these complications in these patients.

Limitations of intentional percutaneous laceration of the anterior mitral leaflet to prevent outflow obstruction

Although LAMPOON is a promising strategy, it requires a high degree of operator skill and a heart team with expertise in electrosurgical techniques and interventional echocardiography. The technique is also limited in patients with a heavily calcified anterior mitral leaflet, although traversal is often possible with careful preprocedural planning, catheter placement, and increased voltage. An essential component of LAMPOON is to ensure the laceration is electrosurgical rather than mechanical. Patients with mechanical splitting of the leaflet are at greatest risk of hemodynamic instability compared with electrical cutting. Given these limitations, the use of LAMPOON is currently relegated to centers of expertise that have an interest/expertise in TMVR.

Mechanical splitting of the anterior leaflet

Although LAMPOON relies on electrosurgical principles to split the AML, work by Lee and colleagues[18] described mechanical splitting of the leaflet. After obtaining transapical access, the anterior leaflet is pierced with a needle, a guidewire is inserted into the right superior pulmonary

artery, and balloon inflation is performed to detach the AML from the mitral annulus. Similar to most techniques for AML modification, this strategy is described only in a case report. Notable limitations are the need for cardiopulmonary bypass and the potential for an inexact splitting of the AML.

Preparation of a U-stitch to correct lateral deflection for endovascular mitral replacement in short landing zone technique

Transcatheter valve-in-valve therapy allows for coaxial deployment of the transcatheter heart valve in the prior surgical valve frame. The lack of such a frame in Valve-in-Ring or Valve-in-MAC therapy make coaxial valve deployment significantly more challenging. The Preparation of a U-stitch to correct Lateral deflection for Endovascular mitral replacement in short landing zone (POULEZ) technique relies on a modification of the Edwards Commander (Edwards Life Science, Irvine, CA) delivery system. A 135-cm-long 3 to 0 polypropylene suture is passed through the catheter nosecone beyond the balloon and through a single petal of the valve pusher. After aligning both along the inner curvature of the delivery system, the distal suture is secured with a knot and the proximal suture is held alongside the delivery handle. TMVR workflow continues in the usual fashion until the valve delivery system crosses the atrial septum. At this stage, the pusher is retracted, creating a fulcrum, and all deflection is removed from the commander delivery system. By placing tension on the free suture end, the valve deflects both medially and anteriorly.[19] This technique may decrease the risk of LVOT obstruction by optimizing coaxiality and appropriate valve placement.

Kissing-balloon technique

A kissing-balloon technique has been used to secure the neo-LVOT. Described in a case report, transesophageal echocardiography was used to guide a 20-mm valvuloplasty balloon into the LVOT. By simultaneously inflating this balloon with transcatheter heart valve deployment, the LVOT was sized and the transcatheter heart valve was optimally oriented.[20] Although this technique is less invasive than others described, it does have significant limitations. Namely, the LVOT balloon does not permanently alter the anterior mitral leaflet increasing the potential risk for LVOT obstruction, and it may increase the likelihood that the transcatheter heart valve is not deployed coaxially.

SUMMARY

TMVR is a promising strategy for patients without options for surgical mitral valve replacement; however, the technique remains limited by a lack of commercially available systems and the risk of LVOT obstruction. This risk can be significantly reduced by detailed CT analysis, procedural planning, and the use of techniques to modify either the anterior mitral leaflet or the interventricular septum. In the future, dedicated devices may make these approaches more efficient, safer, and reproducible.

REFERENCES

1. Regueiro A, Granada JF, Dagenais F, et al. Transcatheter mitral valve replacement: insights from early clinical experience and future challenges. J Am Coll Cardiol 2017;69(17):2175–92.

2. Guerrero M, Urena M, Himbert D, et al. 1-year outcomes of transcatheter mitral valve replacement in patients with severe mitral annular calcification. J Am Coll Cardiol 2018;71(17):1841–53.

3. Kamioka N, Babaliaros V, Morse MA, et al. Comparison of clinical and echocardiographic outcomes after surgical redo mitral valve replacement and transcatheter mitral valve-in-valve therapy. JACC Cardiovasc Interv 2018;11(12):1131–8.

4. Eleid MF, Whisenant BK, Cabalka AK, et al. Percutaneous transvenous transseptal transcatheter valve implantation in failed bioprosthetic mitral valves, ring annuloplasty, and severe mitral annular calcification. JACC Cardiovasc Interv 2016;9(11):1161–74.

5. Blanke P, Dvir D, Cheung A, et al. Mitral annular evaluation with CT in the context of transcatheter mitral valve replacement. JACC Cardiovasc Imaging 2015;8(5):612–5.

6. Babaliaros VC, Greenbaum AB, Khan JM, et al. Intentional percutaneous laceration of the anterior mitral leaflet to prevent outflow obstruction during transcatheter mitral valve replacement: first-in-human experience. JACC Cardiovasc Interv 2017; 10(8):798–809.

7. Khan JM, Greenbaum AB, Khan JM, et al. Intentional laceration of the anterior mitral valve leaflet to prevent left ventricular outflow tract obstruction during transcatheter mitral valve replacement: preclinical findings. JACC Cardiovasc Interv 2016;9(17): 1835–43.

8. Blanke P, Naoum C, Dvir D, et al. Predicting LVOT obstruction in transcatheter mitral valve implantation: concept of the neo-LVOT. JACC Cardiovasc Imaging 2017;10(4):482–5.

9. Wang DD, Eng M, Greenbaum A, et al. Predicting LVOT obstruction after TMVR. JACC Cardiovasc Imaging 2016;9(11):1349–52.

10. Wang DD, Eng MH, Greenbaum AB, et al. Validating a prediction modeling tool for left ventricular outflow tract (LVOT) obstruction after transcatheter mitral valve replacement (TMVR). Catheter Cardiovasc Interv 2018;92(2):379–87.

11. Blanke P, Naoum C, Webb J, et al. Multimodality imaging in the context of transcatheter mitral valve replacement: establishing consensus among modalities and disciplines. JACC Cardiovasc Imaging 2015;8(10):1191–208.

12. David T. Mitral valve replacement with preservation of chorae tendinae: rationale and technical considerations. Ann Thorac Surg 1986;4:680–2.

13. Deharo P, Urena M, Himbert D, et al. Bail-out alcohol septal ablation for left ventricular outflow tract obstruction after transcatheter mitral valve replacement. JACC Cardiovasc Interv 2016;9(8):e73–6.

14. Guerrero M, Wang DD, O'Neill W. Percutaneous alcohol septal ablation to acutely reduce left ventricular outflow tract obstruction induced by transcatheter mitral valve replacement. Catheter Cardiovasc Interv 2016;88(6):E191–7.

15. Guerrero M, Wang DD, Himbert D, et al. Short-term results of alcohol septal ablation as a bail-out strategy to treat severe left ventricular outflow tract obstruction after transcatheter mitral valve replacement in patients with severe mitral annular calcification. Catheter Cardiovasc Interv 2017;90(7):1220–6.

16. Khan JM, Rogers T, Babaliaros VC, et al. Predicting left ventricular outflow tract obstruction despite anterior mitral leaflet resection: the "Skirt NeoLVOT". JACC Cardiovasc Imaging 2018;11(9):1356–9.

17. Greenbaum AB, Condado JF, Eng M, et al. Long or redundant leaflet complicating transcatheter mitral valve replacement: Case vignettes that advocate for removal or reduction of the anterior mitral leaflet. Catheter Cardiovasc Interv 2018;92(3):627–32.

18. Lee R, Hui DS, Helmy TA, et al. Transapical mitral replacement with anterior leaflet splitting: a novel technique to avoid left ventricular outflow tract obstruction. J Thorac Cardiovasc Surg 2018; 155(3):e95–8.

19. Babaliaros V, Greenbaum AB, Kamioka N, et al. Bedside modification of delivery system for transcatheter transseptal mitral replacement with POULEZ system and SAPIEN-3 valve. JACC Cardiovasc Interv 2018;11(12):1207–9.

20. Rahhab Z, Ren B, de Jaegere PPT, et al. Kissing balloon technique to secure the neo-left ventricular outflow tract in transcatheter mitral valve implantation. Eur Heart J 2018;39(23):2220.

Transcatheter Mitral Valve Replacement with Intrepid

Patrick M. McCarthy, MD[a],*, Olga N. Kislitsina, MD, PhD[b], Sukit Chris Malaisrie, MD[c], Charles J. Davidson, MD[d]

KEYWORDS

- Mitral regurgitation • Transcatheter mitral valve replacement • Mitral valve • Apollo trial

KEY POINTS

- The Intrepid valve is a self-expanding nitinol valve that houses a 27-mm trileaflet bovine pericardial valve.
- The diameter of the valve is available in 43-, 46-, or 50-mm diameters.
- Currently, transapical delivery using a 35-French device is available.
- Early feasibility studies and a randomized trial compared with conventional surgery are ongoing.

INTRODUCTION

Mitral regurgitation (MR) can be simply divided into primary (organic) MR caused by leaflet pathologic condition or secondary ("functional") MR secondary to ventricular disease and tethering with "normal" leaflets. Mitral valve replacement (MVR) may be required in some patients with complex primary mitral valve pathologic condition and may be preferred over surgical mitral valve repair in some patients with functional mitral regurgitation (FMR). Surgical MVR is the standard of care[1] but is highly invasive with an elevated mortality compared with repair in most situations. In particular, elderly patients with comorbidities face considerable risk for morbidity and mortality and a difficult recovery after surgery. Transcatheter mitral valve replacement (TMVR) is undergoing early feasibility studies (EFS), and the APOLLO (Transcatheter Mitral Valve Replacement with the Medtronic Intrepid TMVR System in Patients with Severe

Symptomatic Mitral Regurgitation) randomized clinical trial of the use of the Intrepid (Medtronic, Minneapolis, MN) TMVR device versus surgical MVR has commenced.[2–6] This article reviews the key features of the device design, the current implant technique, early clinical results of the EFS, and design of the APOLLO Trial.

THE INTREPID TRANSCATHETER MITRAL VALVE REPLACEMENT SYSTEM

The Intrepid valve was developed by Foundry Newco XII, Inc, which was founded in 2009. The company was later known as Twelve, Inc before being acquired by Medtronic in 2015. The Intrepid valve is based around a size 27-mm trileaflet bovine pericardial valve. This valve is encased in an inner stent frame. The outer frame is available in 3 sizes (43-, 46-, and 50-mm diameters). The self-expanding nitinol system is delivered via a 35-French transapical sheath. The outer frame of the Intrepid valve is

Disclosure Statement: Dr P.M. McCarthy: Edwards Lifescience: consultant and royalties; Abbott Vascular: consultant and advisory board; Medtronic; unpaid member of the Apollo Trial Steering Committee. Dr O.N. Kislitsina: None. Dr S.C. Malaisrie: Edwards Lifescience: consultant, speaker; Medtronic, consultant; Abbott, speaker. Dr C.J. Davidson: Edwards Lifesciences: grant support.

[a] Division of Cardiac Surgery, Northwestern University Feinberg School of Medicine, Northwestern University, 201 East Huron Street, Suite 11-140, Chicago, IL 60611-2908, USA; [b] Cardiology, Northwestern University Feinberg School of Medicine, 201 East Huron Street, Suite 11-140, Chicago, IL 60611-2908, USA; [c] Division of Cardiac Surgery, Northwestern University Feinberg School of Medicine, 201 East Huron Street, Suite 11-140, Chicago, IL 60611, USA; [d] Division of Cardiology, Northwestern University Feinberg School of Medicine, 676 North St. Clair, Arkes 23 Suite 2330, Chicago, IL 60611, USA
* Corresponding author.
E-mail address: Patrick.McCarthy@nm.org

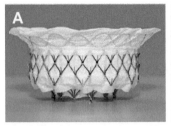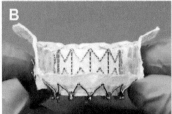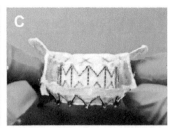

Fig. 1. (*A*) The Intrepid valve is a self-expanding nitinol system delivered via a 35-French transapical sheath. (*B*) Cutouts show the dual stent design. (*C*) Flexibility allows the valve to conform to the mitral annulus shape. (*From* Meredith I, Bapat V, Morriss J, et al. Intrepid transcatheter mitral valve replacement system: technical and product description. EuroIntervention 2016;12(Y):Y78; with permission; and *Courtesy of* Medtronic, Inc, Mounds View, MN.)

flexible, especially the atrial portion, which allows it to conform to the native mitral annulus and the atrial wall (**Fig. 1**). The ventricular portion is stiffer and wider than the native annulus. The distinguishing features of this unique design helps to seat the valve and prevent perivalvular leaks. It is shaped like a champagne cork, and during left ventricular (LV) systole, it is pushed against the annulus, which also minimizes the risk of embolization. Cleats on the outer frame help engage the mitral leaflets and properly seat the valve. The symmetric design allows placement of the valve without having to orient it to the D-shaped mitral annulus.[2]

PROCEDURE PLANNING AND IMPLANT SURGERY

Contrast-enhanced cardiac computed tomography (CT) scan of the mitral annulus is used to determine which size of the prosthesis should be implanted. Proper sizing is based on mitral annular perimeter, intracommissure diameter, septal-lateral diameter, and the potential for LV outflow tract (LVOT) obstruction. The procedure is performed under general anesthesia with guidance by fluoroscopy as well as 2-dimensional (2D) and 3-dimensional (3D) transesophageal echocardiography (TEE; **Fig. 2**). The preprocedure CT scan is used to determine the location of a small left thoracotomy to access the LV apex. The typical location for LV access is to the left of the distal left anterior descending artery. Two purse-string sutures are placed at this location with a tourniquet, which can be tightened around the access sheath. After heparin is given, access is obtained over a guidewire, and the device is advanced through the 35-mm sheath into the mitral annulus (**Fig. 3**). Primarily using TEE, the atrial brim is expanded using a hydraulic delivery mechanism. Fluoroscopy and TEE confirm that it is located above the mitral annulus. The valve is easily manipulated into

the proper orientation relative to the annulus and retracted into the target location in the mitral annulus (**Fig. 4**). The valve is released during a period of rapid ventricular pacing. The delivery system is withdrawn, and the apical sutures are tied during another short burst of rapid pacing and suture reinforced if necessary.

THE INTREPID EARLY FEASIBILITY STUDY

An EFS was designed to determine safety of the TMVR implant. The first operation was performed on May 6, 2015.[3]

The EFS inclusion criteria include symptomatic severe MR; high or extreme surgical risk as determined by the local heart team; mitral valve geometry and size compatible with the available Intrepid sizes; mild or no mitral valve calcification; and an LV ejection fraction greater than or equal to 20%.

Important exclusion criteria include pulmonary hypertension (systolic pressure >70 mm Hg); need for coronary revascularization; hemodynamic instability; need for other valve therapy; renal insufficiency as determined by a serum creatinine greater than 2.5 mg/dL; and prior mitral valve surgery or intervention.

Baseline Characteristics

Fifty consecutive patients (mean age 73 ± 9 years; **Table 1**) were treated with the Intrepid valve as reported by Bapat and colleagues.[3] The mean Society of Thoracic Surgeons (STS) predicted risk of operative mortality was 6.4% ± 5.5% and by the Euro-SCORE was 7.9% ± 6.2%. Eighty-six percent of the patients were New York Heart Association (NYHA) functional class III or IV, and the mean LV ejection fraction was 43%. Most patients had FMR (72%), 16% had primary MR, and 12% had a combination of primary and secondary MR. Forty-five percent of the patients had

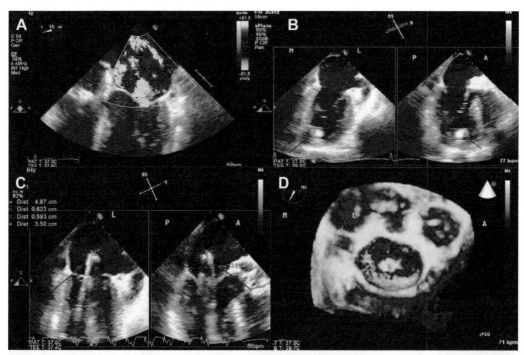

Fig. 2. Implantation of the Intrepid valve. (*A*) Baseline TEE demonstrates severe holosystolic mitral valve regurgitation due to flail leaflets related to myxomatous degenerative disease and fibrocalcific changes (blood pressure = 120/67). (*B*) Following a left thoracotomy, the precise apical access location is confirmed manually (fingertip compression of the LV epicardium) with TEE guidance (*red arrows*). The catheter sheath is placed transapically and the Intrepid valve advanced across the valve into the left atrium (*C, red arrows*) and is centered (*D*) in the MV orifice (surgeon's view).

moderate or severe tricuspid regurgitation. Five patients had functioning aortic valve prostheses.

Procedural Results

Of the 50 patients, 1 patient did not undergo implantation because of bleeding from the LV apex. Of the 49 patients with attempted TMVR, a successful implant was achieved in 48 (98%), with a median overall procedure time of 100 minutes (interquartile range [IQR], 80 to 124 minutes). The median time for device deployment was 14 minutes (IQR, 12–17 minutes). The failure to implant was related to a sizing miscalculation and malpositioning of the valve. There was no incidence of device malfunction, failure, or need for open cardiac surgery. Mechanical support with an intra-aortic balloon pump was used in 5 patients (2 prophylactically, and 3 for hemodynamic management), and with extracorporeal membrane oxygenation in 3 patients (1 for worsening pulmonary hypertension, and 2 to assist in bleeding control from the LV apex).

Clinical Outcomes

Thirty-day mortality occurred in 7 patients (14%). Three deaths were related to LV apical bleeding during or shortly after the procedure, including 1

patient with valve malposition. Three other patients died of heart failure within 30 days after the procedure. The median clinical follow-up for the entire cohort was 173 days (IQR, 54–342 days) (Fig. 5). Four additional patients died after 30 days (between days 54 and 122), but there were no deaths after 4 months. Three of the late deaths were caused by sudden cardiac arrest, and 1 death wase caused by intracranial hemorrhage following a fall. In the cases of all late deaths, absence of structural valve deterioration was documented at autopsy or with echocardiography within the prior month before death.

Reduction in Mitral Regurgitation

Preoperative MR was severe in 47 patients (95.9%) and moderate in 2 patients. Postimplant MR was zero in 74% and mild in 26% (periprosthetic in 3 patients, and prosthetic in 8 patients). The results of MR reduction were sustained beyond 30 days with no new mild or greater MR, and no patients had MR greater than mild. After implant, there was no evidence of LVOT obstruction or mitral stenosis (mean gradient across the valve was 4.1 ± 1.3 mm Hg). NYHA class and quality of life also improved over follow-up (Fig. 6).

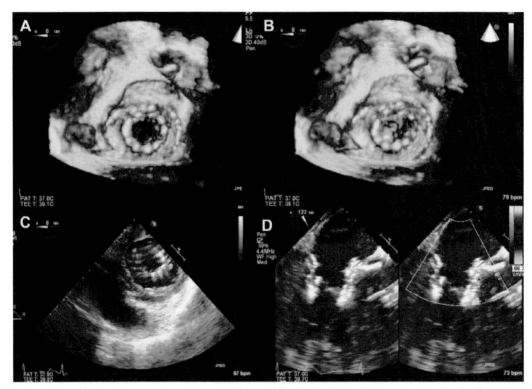

Fig. 3. After confirming the correct positioning of the valve (in relationship to the anatomic landmarks, typically the coronary sinus and left circumflex artery), the valve was gradually opened in the left atrium above the annulus. Then, the valve was retracted to the preplanned landmarks, and with rapid pacing, the valve was released in the mitral annulus and valve without complication. (A, B) 3D "surgeons view" of the mitral valve open and closed, (C) 2D TEE demonstrates complete deployment, and (D) color flow imaging shows the TMVR was successfully deployed with a mean gradient 3 mm Hg and trivial valvular and paravalvular (posterior) regurgitation (blood pressure, 100/70).

THE APOLLO PIVOTAL TRIAL

The APOLLO Trial commenced in 2018 (Clinical-Trials.gov [4] identifier, #NCT03242642) as a randomized clinical trial comparing the Intrepid valve implant with conventional mitral surgery (anticipated MVR), and with a single-arm cohort for patients who are judged ineligible for surgery

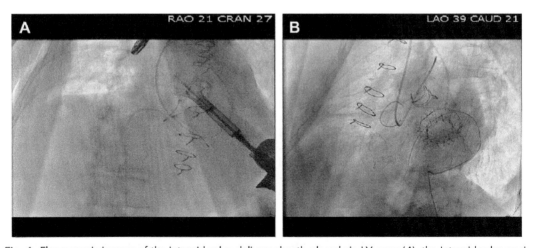

Fig. 4. Fluoroscopic images of the Intrepid valve delivery sheath placed via LV apex (A), the Intrepid valve positioned across the mitral valve, and (B) the successfully deployed valve (note there had been prior aortic valve replacement and tricuspid ring surgery).

Table 1
Select characteristics of patients in early feasibility trial

Baseline Characteristics (N = 50)	
Age, y	72.6 ± 9.4
Men	29 (58)
New York Heart Association functional class	
II	7 (14.0)
III	35 (70.0)
IV	8 (16.0)
Heart failure hospitalization within past year (≥1)	29 (58.0)
Chronic obstructive pulmonary disease	25 (50.0)
Chronic renal insufficiency	29 (58.0)
Glomerular filtration rate, 30–60 mL/min/m²	25 (50.0)
Atrial fibrillation	29 (58.0)
Prior stroke	8 (16.0)
Coronary artery disease	34 (68.0)
Prior myocardial infarction	22 (44.0)
Mild or worse mitral annular calcification	17 (34.0)
Number of sternotomies ≥1	22 (44.0)
Prior coronary artery bypass surgery	19 (38.0)
Extenuating circumstances	
Frailty	16 (32.0)
Pulmonary hypertension	20 (40.0)
Poor mobility	7 (14.0)
Albumin <3.3 g/dL	9 (23.1)
Anemia	22 (44.0)
Liver dysfunction	4 (9.5)
Malignancy	15 (30.0)
Immunosuppression	2.0 (4.0)

Values are mean ± standard deviation or n (%).
From Bapat V, Rajagopal V, Meduri C, et al. Early experience with new transcatheter mitral valve replacement. J Am Coll Cardiol 2018;71(1):16; with permission.

(Fig. 7). It is anticipated that 1380 patients will be recruited. Key aspects of the trial are summarized in later discussion.

The primary endpoint is a composite of all-cause mortality, all stroke, reoperation (or reintervention), and cardiovascular hospitalization at 1-year follow-up. Secondary endpoints include the composite of all-cause mortality, disabling stroke, acute kidney injury, prolonged ventilation, deep wound infection, reoperation

(or reintervention) for any reason, and major bleeding at 30 days or hospital discharge, whichever is later; change in NYHA class at 1 year; quality-of-life improvement at 30 days as measured by Short Form-12 Health Survey and at 1 year as measured by the Kansas City Cardiovascular Questionnaire; echocardiographic assessments of degree of MR as measured by echocardiography at 1 year; days alive out of hospital (all hospitalizations) at 1 year; and cardiovascular hospitalizations at 1 year.

Key inclusion criteria for enrollment in the trial include moderate to severe or severe MR (per American Society of Echocardiography 2017 Guidelines and Standards definition) and for the patient to be a candidate for bioprosthetic MVR, as determined by the heart team. Key exclusion criteria include prior transcatheter mitral valve procedure with device currently implanted; anatomic contraindications; prohibitive mitral annular calcification; LV ejection fraction less than 25%; need for emergent or urgent surgery; and hemodynamic instability.

Patients with predicted risk of operative mortality ≥3% or less than 35% risk of mortality or irreversible major morbidity at 30 days will be entered into the randomized arms of the trial (TMVR or conventional mitral valve surgery), whereas patients who are ineligible for conventional mitral valve surgery based on predicted risk of ≥35% and less than 50% of mortality or irreversible major morbidity will be enrolled in the observational, single-arm cohort and undergo TMVR.

DISCUSSION
Lessons Learned from the Early Feasibility Study

The EFS study confirmed that this was a sick patient population with approximately 6.4% predicted risk of operative mortality per STS score and 8% per EuroSCORE II. Device implant was successful in 48/50 patients (49/50 in whom it was introduced into the LV) in this earliest experience and is facilitated by good imaging. High-quality imaging to guide placement, performed by experienced echocardiographers, is of paramount importance. Also, clear and open communication between the operator and echocardiographer makes the procedure progress smoothly as evidenced by the implant time of only 14 minutes. The anesthesiologist is a key partner because cardiac output may drop with rapid pacing in these impaired ventricles, and hemodynamic instability or LVOT obstruction may follow device implantation. Preprocedural planning with all members of the team is critical

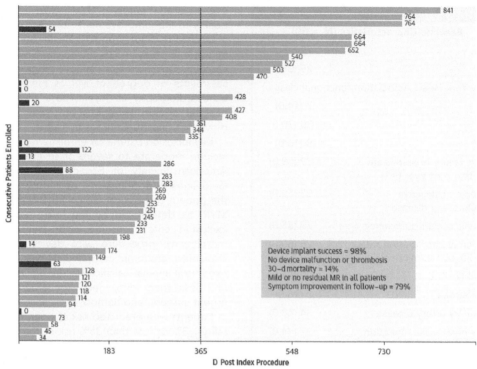

CENTRAL ILLUSTRATION Early Clinical Experience of TMVR with the New Valve Prosthesis

(Chart y-axis: Consecutive Patients Enrolled; x-axis: D Post Index Procedure, with gridlines at 183, 365, 548, 730)

Inset text:
Device implant success = 98%
No device malfunction or thrombosis
30-d mortality = 14%
Mild or no residual MR in all patients
Symptom improvement in follow-up = 79%

Fig. 5. Summary of early follow-up and outcomes for consecutive patients enrolled in an EFS enrolling patients in Australia, Europe, and the United States. Follow-up time for the 50 patients is illustrated with patients listed on the y-axis in descending order of treatment. X-axis indicates duration of follow-up. All deaths occurred before 365 days (dotted line). Blue, surviving patients; orange, deceased patients. (*From* Bapat V, Rajagopal V, Meduri C, et al. Early experience with new transcatheter mitral valve replacement. J Am Coll Cardiol 2018;71(1):17; with permission.)

to prepare for all possibilities and options for treatment of complications.

There was an unexpected number of transapical complications and bleeding in the EFS that led to adverse events and death (6% of the group died of apical access bleeding). Although transapical transcatheter aortic valve replacement (TAVR) has also been occasionally plagued with this complication, it occurs much less frequently than reported here; this may in part be due to the larger sheaths currently required for first-generation TMVR devices.[7] In the case of transapical TAVR, perhaps the ventricular hypertrophy related to the aortic stenosis is somewhat protective in this regard. Some of the apical bleeding did not occur immediately at the time of implant, but was delayed, and implies that careful vigilance of the patient and blood pressure management postoperatively should be mandatory. Perhaps the use of a transapical closure device, such as a duct occluder, could mitigate this problem. Also, careful imaging of the LV apex and left pleural space to assess the possible accumulation of

blood, including the late development of a pseudoaneurysm, should be part of the routine follow-up.

Potential LVOT obstruction was carefully assessed before implantation and led to several patients determined not to be candidates for implant because of a predicted high LVOT gradient in the neo-LVOT. Indeed, in the EFS series there were no LVOT obstructions observed, indicating that the selection was perhaps overly cautious. By design, the Intrepid device projects only approximately 18 mm into the ventricular side of the mitral annulus, not much different than most surgically implanted bioprostheses. As experience develops, the authors will be able to better predict which patients may be at risk for neo-LVOT obstruction and how the orientation of the valve (eg, toward the septum) may impact this.

Management of Low Ejection Fraction and Hemodynamic Instability

Many of the patients with FMR also have heart failure (86% NYHA FC III or IV). At Northwestern,

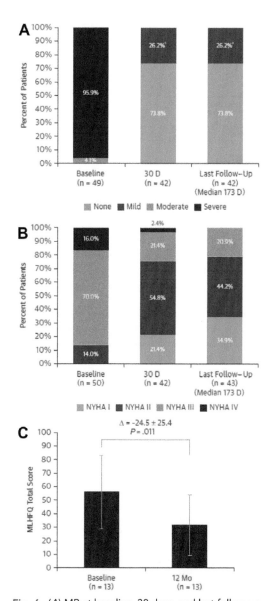

Fig. 6. (A) MR at baseline, 30 days, and last follow-up. (B) NHYA functional class at baseline, 30 days, and last follow-up. (C) Minnesota Living With Heart Failure Questionnaire total score at baseline and 1 year. [a] Three patients (7.1%) had mild paravalvular MR, and 8 patients (19.0%) had mild transvalvular MR graded. MLHFQ, Minnesota Living with Heart Failure Questionnaire. (*From* Bapat V, Rajagopal V, Meduri C, et al. Early experience with new transcatheter mitral valve replacement. J Am Coll Cardiol 2018;71(1):19; with permission.)

the heart failure team is consulted preoperatively to manage patients with FMR and/or a history of heart failure. The heart failure team (including nurse practitioners) optimizes the medical condition before surgery by adjusting medications and carefully monitoring the patient perioperatively and after discharge. The Cardio-MEMs device[8] (Abbott Laboratories, Abbott

Park, IL) is implanted in select patients to provide excellent data for perioperative and long-term management. With this, they have been able to ensure that patients are euvolemic on the day of surgery. After the patient leaves the intensive care unit, monitoring of pulmonary artery pressures for adjustment of diuretics and other medications can continue on the regular nursing floor. It also has helped keep patients out of the hospital after discharge. Perioperatively in the EFS study, several patients received an intra-aortic balloon pump or extracorporeal membrane oxygenation. In the Northwestern experience with surgery for heart failure patients, the focus in on the optimization of preload, afterload, and inotropes to avoid mechanical support that can slow down recovery.[9]

Patients Selection for Transcatheter Mitral Valve Replacement

The recently published Clinical Outcomes Assessment of the MitraClip Percutaneous Therapy for High Surgical Risk Patients (COAPT) trial[10] demonstrates that patients with FMR are a target population for therapy in that a subset of these patients will have improved outcomes with a reduction of MR. TMVR may be preferred in those patients who were not anatomic candidates for a leaflet approach using a clip device or investigational transcatheter annular reduction devices. Many patients, however, especially older patients and patients with comorbidities, may have a combination of FMR as well as some aspect of prolapse. In addition, some patients with degenerative MR may have very complex disease with calcification of the leaflets that is not amenable to reliable surgical repair and would be better served with an MVR. The optimal patient population for TMVR is not yet fully established. The MitraClip (Abbott Laboratories, Abbott Park, IL) experience with the COAPT trial only occurred after tens of thousands had been treated, including many patients with FMR who were being treated in Europe. Nevertheless, some patients will be excellent candidates for TMVR as opposed to an open surgical approach, and the APOLLO trial will help us to better understand this population.

APOLLO Trial

The APOLLO trial recently commenced and has an aggressive enrollment target of a maximum of 1380 patients. New criteria in development to determine anatomic eligibility based on prediction of the postimplantation neo-LVOT area should help facilitate enrollment. This trial is a complex trial, and a lesson learned from the

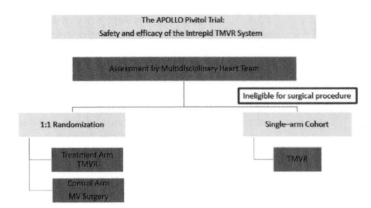

Fig. 7. Flow diagram for the APOLLO trial enrollment.

COAPT trial would be the importance of guideline-directed medical therapy for the patients who have heart failure. In the COAPT trial, the outcomes were remarkably better than in the MITRA-FR (Multicentre Study of Percutaneous Mitral Valve Repair MitraClip Device in Patients With Severe Secondary Mitral Regurgitation) trial.[10,11] It is thought that the rigorous focus on guideline-directed medical therapy in COAPT, as opposed to the "real-world" non-protocolized approach to medical therapy used in Mitra-FR, may have played a significant role in achieving the excellent long-term outcomes observed in COAPT patients treated with MitraClip.

SUMMARY

TMVR with the Intrepid device is a promising approach for patients who need MVR and who are moderate to prohibitive risk for surgery. Further iterations of the Intrepid valve include retrievability, which is a hallmark of self-expandable valves. In addition, a transfemoral venous approach with transseptal/transatrial access will be welcome and will likely decrease the complications that have been observed with transapical implants. However, the pace of improvements will not be as rapid as with TAVR. The variability in mitral valve anatomy, pathophysiology, and postimplant physiology is very different from aortic stenosis patients treated with TAVR, and these factors present a far greater challenge for TMVR implants.

REFERENCES

1. Nishimura RA, Otto CM, Bonow RO, et al. 2017 AHA/ACC focused update of the 2014 AHA/ACC guideline for the management of patients with valvular heart disease: a report of the American College of Cardiology/American Heart Association Task Force on clinical practice guidelines. Circulation 2017;135(25):e1159–95.

2. Meredith I, Bapat V, Morriss J, et al. Intrepid transcatheter mitral valve replacement system: technical and product description. EuroIntervention 2016;12(Y):Y78–80.

3. Bapat V, Rajagopal V, Meduri C, et al. Early experience with new transcatheter mitral valve replacement. J Am Coll Cardiol 2018;71(1):12–21.

4. Transcatheter mitral valve replacement with the medtronic intrepid™ TMVR system in patients with severe symptomatic mitral regurgitation (APOLLO). Available at: https://clinicaltrials.gov/ct2/show/study/NCT03242642?term=intrepid&rank=3&show_locs=Y#locn. Accessed December 14, 2018.

5. Tang GH, George I, Hahn RT, et al. Transcatheter mitral valve replacement: design implications, potential pitfalls and outcomes assessment. Cardiol Rev 2015;23(6):290–6.

6. Sorajja P, Bapat V. Early experience with the Intrepid system for transcatheter mitral valve replacement. Ann Cardiothorac Surg 2018;7(6):792–8.

7. Wyler von Ballmoos MC, Kalra A, Reardon MJ. Complexities of transcatheter mitral valve replacement (TMVR) and why it is not transcatheter aortic valve replacement (TAVR). Ann Cardiothorac Surg 2018;7(6):724–30.

8. Heywood JT, Jermyn R, Shavelle D, et al. Impact of practice-based management of pulmonary artery pressures in 2000 patients implanted with the CardioMEMS sensor. Circulation 2017;135(16):1509–17.

9. McCarthy PM. Valve surgery for patients with left ventricular dysfunction. In: McCarthy PM, Young JB, editors. Heart failure: a combined medical and surgical approach. Malden (MA): Blackwell Futura; 2007. p. 153–73.

10. Obadia JF, Messika-Zeitoun D, Leurent G, et al. Percutaneous repair or medical treatment for secondary mitral regurgitation. N Engl J Med 2018;379:2297–306.

11. Stone GW, Lindenfeld J, Abraham WT, et al. Transcatheter mitral-valve repair in patients with heart failure. N Engl J Med 2018;379:2307–18.

Transcatheter Mitral Valve Replacement with Tendyne

Hiroki Niikura, MD[a], Mario Gössl, MD, PhD[a], Paul Sorajja, MD[b],*

KEYWORDS

- Mitral regurgitation • Transcatheter mitral valve replacement • Tendyne valve prosthesis

KEY POINTS

- The Tendyne valve (Abbott Structural, Santa Clara, CA) is a self-expanding, retrievable, and repositionable nitinol prothesis with a double-frame design that is delivered via a 34F transapical sheath and uniquely anchored with a tether connected to an epicardial hemostatic pad at the apex.
- Patient evaluation relies on a heart team evaluation and multimodality imaging to determine the mitral regurgitation (MR) severity and mechanism, degree of mitral annular calcification, angulation of the aortic-mitral curtain, left ventricular outflow tract (LVOT) size, elongation or tethering of the mitral valve (MV) leaflets, presence of systolic anterior motion of the anterior mitral leaflet, and potential for LVOT obstruction after implantation.
- The Tendyne Global Feasibility Study demonstrated acceptable procedural safety (no procedural deaths), with durable reduction in MR, reduction in left ventricular volumes, and improvement in quality of life at 30-day and 1-year follow-ups.
- SUMMIT (Clinical Trial to Evaluate the Safety and Effectiveness of Using the Tendyne Mitral Valve System for the Treatment of Symptomatic Mitral Regurgitation) is the pivotal clinical trial of the Tendyne valve in the United States and randomly assigns patients with severe MR to either conventional MV surgery or transcatheter mitral valve replacement (TMVR) with the Tendyne valve; patients who fulfill the inclusion and exclusion criteria but are ineligible for surgery or transcatheter edge-to-edge repair will receive the TMVR with the Tendyne valve as part of a single-arm cohort.

INTRODUCTION

Mitral regurgitation (MR) is the most commonly occurring valvular heart disease in developed countries, with approximately 3.5 million people in the United States having above moderate-to-severe MR. Among those over 75 years of age, the prevalence of MR is greater than 10%, and the incidence of MR is expected to increase due to population aging.[1,2] The mitral valve (MV) apparatus is a complex structure with disease related to primary causes (ie, abnormality of the MV apparatus) or secondary causes (ie, annular dilation and leaflet tethering due to disease of the left atrium [LA] or left ventricle [LV]). Whether primary or secondary, severe MR carries an adverse prognosis, with a survival comparable to or even worse than that of most advanced malignancies.[3–5] Surgical repair or replacement is the gold standard therapy for patients with symptomatic MR, whereas transcatheter edge-to-edge repair with MitraClip (Abbott Structural, Santa Clara, California) has proved of clinical benefit in selected patients. This article

Disclosures: P. Sorajja: Medtronic: consulting, speaking, and research grants; Edwards Lifesciences: consulting, speaking, and research grants; Boston Scientific: consulting, speaking, and research grants; Pipeline: consulting and equity; Admedus: consulting and equity; and Abbott Structural: consulting, speaking, and research grants. All other authors have no disclosures.
[a] Valve Science Center, Minneapolis Heart Institute Foundation, Abbott Northwestern Hospital, 920 East 28th Street, Minneapolis, MN 55407, USA; [b] Valve Science Center, Minneapolis Heart Institute Foundation, Abbott Northwestern Hospital, 920 East 28th Street, Suite 200, Minneapolis, MN 55407, USA
* Corresponding author.
E-mail address: paul.sorajja@allina.com

discusses the potential role for transcatheter MV replacement (TMVR) with the Tendyne valve (Abbott Structural, Santa Clara, California).

THE TENDYNE VALVE PROSTHESIS

The Tendyne valve is a self-expanding, nitinol prothesis with a double-frame design that contains a trileaflet porcine pericardial valve and has an effective orifice area of greater than 3.2 cm^2 (standard size) or 2.0 cm^2 (low profile size). The prosthesis is anatomically shaped for the mitral annulus. The outer frame contains a cuff that extends above the plane of the annulus to abut the anterior atrial wall and aortic-mitral continuity for the purposes of preventing diastolic paravalvular MR. The size of the outer frame ranges from 30 mm to 43 mm in the septal-lateral dimension and 34 mm to 50 mm in the intercommissural dimension. Implanted valves are selected to be larger than native mitral orifice. The prosthesis, which is delivered via a 34F transapical sheath, is uniquely anchored with a tether connected to an epicardial hemostatic pad at the apex (Fig. 1). The Tendyne prosthesis is retrievable and repositionable after full deployment, an ability that minimizes the need for bailout open surgery.

PATIENT SELECTION

Patient evaluation by a multidisciplinary heart team is paramount to optimize procedural results and effectiveness of TMVR. The Tendyne Global Feasibility Study (ClinicalTrials.gov identifier, NCT02321514) enrolled patients with symptomatic (New York Heart Association [NYHA] functional class ≥II) grade 3 or grade 4 degenerative or functional MR. Key exclusion criteria included LV end-diastolic diameter greater than 70 mm, severe mitral annular or leaflet calcification, LA thrombus or LV thrombus, prior mitral or aortic valve surgery or intervention, pulmonary artery systolic pressure greater than or equal to 70 mm Hg, severe tricuspid regurgitation, and severe right ventricular dysfunction.[6]

All patients considered for TMVR underwent preprocedural multimodality imaging with transthoracic echocardiography, transesophageal echocardiography (TEE), and contrast-enhanced, gated-cardiac CT. These evaluations determine the severity and mechanism of MR, MV morphology, degree of mitral annular calcification (MAC), angulation of the aortic-mitral curtain, LV outflow tract (LVOT) size, LV dilatation, elongation or tethering of the MV leaflets, and the presence of systolic anterior motion (SAM) of the anterior mitral leaflet (AML). Using cardiac CT, measurements with prosthesis overlay for mitral annular sizing, fit, identification of the LV myocardial entry site, and the potential for LVOT obstruction (ie, calculation of the neo-LVOT area) were performed.[6–9] Strict criteria for neo-LVOT area measurements were not applied, but general cutoff values of 150 mm^2 and 250 mm^2 during systole were used.

TECHNIQUE FOR DEPLOYMENT

The deployment procedure is performed under general anesthesia using a transapical approach via a left minithoracotomy. The site for LV apical access that bisects the MV in both the commissural and septal-lateral planes is determined by the preprocedural CT and intraprocedural TEE. The myocardial access site is punctured with a multipurpose needle, followed by placement of a standard 7F sheath. A balloon-tip catheter is advanced from the LV into the LA, with care to avoid chordal entanglement, which is confirmed with TEE. A 36F delivery sheath is inserted into the LV over a 0.035-inch guide wire. The atrial cuff of the Tendyne prosthesis is extruded and then rotated to fit the anatomic shape of the native MV using TEE. The prosthesis is withdrawn toward the LV and deployed intra-annularly. After deployment, anchoring is achieved by a tether connected to an epicardial pad, which also provides hemostasis. The tension and length from the valve to the ventricular apex of the tether are adjusted after deployment to optimize the seating of the prosthesis without worsening of LV filling pressures (ie, LV end-diastolic pressure). If the function of the prosthesis is not acceptable, or if LVOT obstruction occurs, the prosthesis can be repositioned or fully retrieved (Fig. 2). The entire procedure is performed without cardiopulmonary bypass and without rapid ventricular pacing.[6,10] Optimal antithrombotic therapeutic regimens of antiplatelet and anticoagulant therapy in patients who underwent Tendyne valve implantation have not been established, but antiplatelet therapy with aspirin (81–100 mg daily) or clopidogrel (75 mg daily) and anticoagulant therapy with heparin, followed by warfarin for greater than or equal to 3 months, with a target international normalized ratio of 2.5 to 3.5, in general, were used.[6]

CLINICAL OUTCOMES

The Tendyne Global Feasibility Study was a prospective, open-label, nonrandomized trial to establish the safety and efficacy of the Tendyne

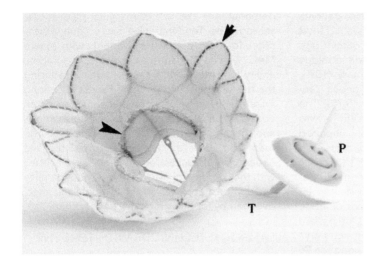

Fig. 1. The Tendyne MV system. The nitinol self-expanding prosthesis has a double flame. An outer flame (*arrow*) contains a cuff and an inner flame has a trileaflet porcine pericardial valve (*arrowhead*). The prosthesis is anchored to an epicardial hemostatic pad (P) by a tether (T). (*Courtesy of* Abbott, Inc., Santa Clara, CA; with permission.)

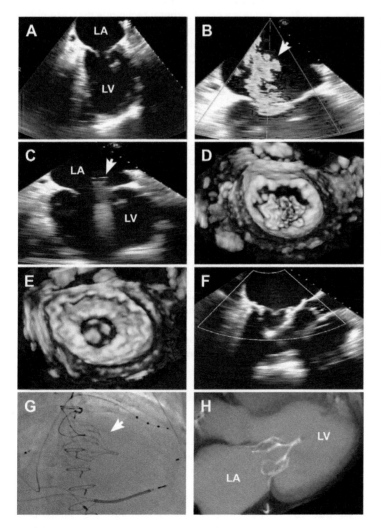

Fig. 2. Transcatheter MV implantation with Tendyne valve. (*A, B*) TEE showing severe secondary MR (*arrow*). (*C*) The 34F Tendyne sheath (*arrow*) with the prosthesis was advanced into position transapically and centered in the MV orifice using TEE guidance. (*D*) The Tendyne prosthesis was partially extruded in the LA on 3-D TEE imaging. (*E*) The Tendyne prosthesis aligned anatomically and then fully extruded in the LA on 3-D TEE imaging. (*F*) Doppler color-flow imaging shows no residual MR. (*G*) Fluoroscopy demonstrating placement of the Tendyne prosthesis (*arrow*). (*H*) CT demonstrating the Tendyne prosthesis in LVOT view.

valve at 30-day follow-up.[6] A total of 30 patients with grade 3 or grade 4 MR underwent TMVR using the Tendyne valve. The mean patient age was 75.6 years ± 9.2 years. The MR etiology was either secondary (76%) or primary (10%). The mean Society of Thoracic Surgeons predicted risk of mortality was 7.3% ± 5.7%. The mean LV ejection fraction (LVEF) was 47.1% ± 9.2% and was moderately impaired (LVEF 30% to 50%) in 48.3% of patients and severely impaired (LVEF <30%) in 10.3%. Device implantation was successful in 28 of the 30 patients (93.3%) without procedural death, in-hospital stroke, myocardial infarction, or additional device-related complications. One patient died 13 days postoperatively due to pneumonia and respiratory failure. At 30 days, among the 26 surviving patients receiving the Tendyne valve who underwent transthoracic echocardiography imaging, MR was absent in 25 patients and mild in 1 patient. The LV end-diastolic volume index significantly decreased (90.1 mL/m^2 ± 19.7 mL/m^2 at baseline vs 72.1 mL/m^2 ± 19.3 mL/m^2 at follow-up; P = .0012). A total of 21 patients (75%) demonstrated mild or no symptoms (NYHA I or II) at follow-up. One patient, whose anticoagulation was subtherapeutic, had evidence of leaflet thrombosis on CT imaging. The rate of successful valve implantation free of cardiovascular mortality, stroke, and device malfunction was 86.6% at 30 days.

Sorajja[11] reported long-term results from the first 100 patients enrolled in the Global Feasibility Study. Mean age was 75.4 years ± 8.1 years and all patients had grade 3 or grade 4 MR, with a majority of patients (90%) having secondary MR. The mean Society of Thoracic Surgeons predicted risk of operative mortality was 7.9% ± 5.7% and the mean LVEF was 46.4% ± 9.6%. Successful valve implantation occurred in 97% of patients without procedural death, stroke, or conversions to cardiac surgery; 30-day mortality was 6% and the rate of 1-year survival was 72%. At 1 year, durable elimination of MR was demonstrated in 98% of patients, 86.5% of survivors were NYHA I or II, and 78% of survivors showed improved quality-of-life, with the Kansas City Cardiomyopathy Questionnaire (KCCQ) scores increased greater than 5 points.

USE IN SEVERE MITRAL ANNULAR CALCIFICATION

Severe MAC is a high-risk condition in which surgery may be prohibitive due to the potential for fatal atrioventricular groove disruption. Transcatheter options are severely limited due to the risk of LVOT obstruction, embolization potential, and the risk of marginal paravalvular sealing. The Tendyne valve has unique advantages for the treatment of patients with severe MAC, with its D-shaped anatomic configuration, ability to retrieve and be repositioned (reducing the risk of LVOT obstruction), robust anchoring system consisting of a tether connected to an epicardial pad (reducing the risk of embolization), and sealing skirts (reducing paravalvular regurgitation). In 2017, the authors reported the first experience of successful TMVR for severe MAC with the compassionate use of the Tendyne valve and demonstrated the feasibility of safe and effective therapy for these high-risk patients (Fig. 3).[12]

LAMPOON TECHNIQUE WITH TENDYNE

TMVR may cause fatal LVOT obstruction due to septal displacement of the AML and obstruction from SAM of the AML. The laceration of the AML to prevent LVOT obstruction (LAMPOON) technique is a novel catheter technique that resembles surgical chord-sparing AML resection and may enable the deployment of TMVR in patients with high risk of LVOT obstruction. This technique resembles David's[13] surgical anterior resection with chordal sparing. Recently, Khan and colleagues[14] reported the first experience of successfully using the LAMPOON technique with the Tendyne valve to prevent LVOT obstruction due to SAM. This technique may expand the options available for patients who can benefit from TMVR.

CLINICAL TRIALS
Global Feasibility Study
The Global Feasibility Study is a single-arm, multicenter feasibility study. The aim is to examine early and long-term clinical outcomes of TMVR with the Tendyne valve (including compassionate use) in patients with high or prohibitive surgical risk. This study will enroll up to 350 patients who have either primary MR or secondary MR in the United States, European Union, and Australia. The primary safety and performance endpoints are device success and freedom from device-related or procedure-related serious adverse events at 30 days. The efficacy endpoints include rehospitalization or reintervention for heart failure, change in NYHA functional class, and quality-of-life with KCCQ score at 1 year (Expanded Clinical Study of the Tendyne Mitral Valve System ClinicalTrials.gov identifier, NCT02321514).

The SUMMIT Trial
The Clinical Trial to Evaluate the Safety and Effectiveness of Using the Tendyne Mitral Valve

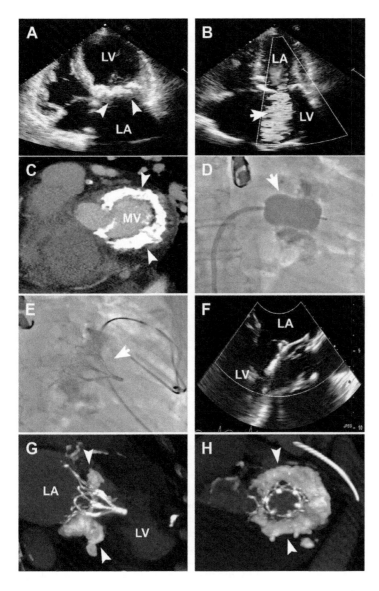

Fig. 3. Transcatheter MV implantation with Tendyne valve in severe MAC. (*A*) TEE showing severe MAC (*arrowheads*). (*B*) TEE showing severe secondary MR (*arrow*). (*C*) Preprocedural CT demonstrating a large severe MAC on the MV (*arrowheads*). (*D*) Fluoroscopy demonstrating predilatation with balloon valvuloplasty (*arrow*). (*E*) Fluoroscopy demonstrating placement of the Tendyne prosthesis (*arrow*). (*F*) Doppler color-flow imaging shows no residual MR. (*G, H*) Postprocedural CT demonstrating fitting the Tendyne prosthesis within the severe MAC (*arrowheads*).

System for the Treatment of Symptomatic Mitral Regurgitation (SUMMIT) is the pivotal clinical trial of the TMVR with the Tendyne valve in the United States. This trial will enroll up to 1010 patients at 80 sites in the United States, European Union, and Canada. The trial design has a surgical arm and a nonsurgical arm. Subjects in the surgical arm will be randomized in a 2:1 ratio to the trial device or to conventional surgery, which consist of either replacement or repair. Subjects in the nonsurgical arm must be ineligible for edge-to-edge repair with the MitraClip and receive the Tendyne valve as part of an observational registry. The primary endpoint in both cohorts of the trial is a composite endpoint

of death, cardiovascular hospitalization, stroke, or reoperation at 1 year (Clinical Trial to Evaluate the Safety and Effectiveness of Using the Tendyne Mitral Valve System for the Treatment of Symptomatic Mitral Regurgitation (SUMMIT) ClinicalTrials.gov identifier, NCT03433274).

The Tendyne Mitral Annular Calcification Study

An early feasibility study of the Tendyne valve for use in subjects with symptomatic, severe MR and severe MAC is currently recruiting patients. The Tendyne MAC study is a single-arm, multicenter feasibility study that plans to include up to 30 patients at no more than 10 centers, with a focus on patients not suitable for conventional surgery. The primary endpoint is procedural success, defined as successful device implantation and freedom from serious device-related and procedure-related adverse events at 30-day follow-up (Feasibility Study of the Tendyne Mitral Valve System for Use in Subjects With Mitral Annular Calcification ClinicalTrials.gov identifier, NCT03539458).

SUMMARY

TMVR has emerged as a novel potential therapy for patients with severe MV disease who are unsuitable candidates for conventional surgery and transcatheter mitral repair with MitraClip. Although the field of TMVR is still in its infancy, TMVR with the Tendyne valve has shown potential as an effective and safe treatment alternative for high-risk patients with severe MV disease at short-term follow-up. Further ongoing studies ultimately will determine its role in the management of patients with MR.

REFERENCES

1. Nkomo VT, Gardin JM, Skelton TN, et al. Burden of valvular heart diseases: a population-based study. Lancet 2006;368(9540):1005–11.
2. Coffey S, Cairns BJ, Iung B. The modern epidemiology of heart valve disease. Heart 2016;102(1): 75–85.
3. Enriquez-Sarano M, Avierinos JF, Messika-Zeitoun D, et al. Quantitative determinants of the outcome of asymptomatic mitral regurgitation. N Engl J Med 2005;352(9):875–83.
4. Rossi A, Zoppini G, Benfari G, et al. Mitral regurgitation and increased risk of all-cause and cardiovascular mortality in patients with type 2 diabetes. Am J Med 2017;130(1):70–6.e1.
5. Grigioni F, Enriquez-Sarano M, Zehr KJ, et al. Ischemic mitral regurgitation: long-term outcome and prognostic implications with quantitative Doppler assessment. Circulation 2001;103(13): 1759–64.
6. Muller DW, Farivar RS, Jansz P, et al. Transcatheter mitral valve replacement for patients with symptomatic mitral regurgitation: a global feasibility trial. J Am Coll Cardiol 2017;69(4):381–91.
7. Blanke P, Naoum C, Dvir D, et al. Predicting LVOT obstruction in transcatheter mitral valve implantation: concept of the neo-LVOT. JACC Cardiovasc Imaging 2017;10(4):482–5.
8. Naoum C, Leipsic J, Cheung A, et al. Mitral annular dimensions and geometry in patients with functional mitral regurgitation and mitral valve prolapse: implications for transcatheter mitral valve implantation. JACC Cardiovasc Imaging 2016;9(3): 269–80.
9. Abdelghani M, Spitzer E, Soliman OII, et al. A simplified and reproducible method to size the mitral annulus: implications for transcatheter mitral valve replacement. Eur Heart J Cardiovasc Imaging 2017;18(6):697–706.
10. Regueiro A, Granada JF, Dagenais F, et al. Transcatheter mitral valve replacement: insights from early clinical experience and future challenges. J Am Coll Cardiol 2017;69(17):2175–92.
11. Sorajja P. Key note intervention studies: TENDYNE transcatheter mitral prosthesis: long-term results from the first 100 patients enrolled in the global feasibility study. San Diego (CA): TCT 2018; 2018.
12. Sorajja P, Gossl M, Bae R, et al. Severe mitral annular calcification: first experience with transcatheter therapy using a dedicated mitral prosthesis. JACC Cardiovasc Interv 2017;10(11):1178–9.
13. David TE. Mitral valve replacement with preservation of chordae tendinae: rationale and technical considerations. Ann Thorac Surg 1986;41(6):680–2.
14. Khan JM, Lederman RJ, Devireddy CM, et al. LAMPOON to facilitate tendyne transcatheter mitral valve replacement. JACC Cardiovasc Interv 2018;11(19):2014–7.

Transcatheter Mitral Valve Replacement in Patients with Severe Mitral Annular Calcification

Sung-Han Yoon, MD, Raj Makkar, MD*

KEYWORDS

• Aortic stenosis • Transcatheter aortic valve implantation • Bicuspid aortic valve

KEY POINTS

- Mitral annular calcification (MAC) is a fibrous, degenerative calcification of the mitral valve, and patients with severe MAC associated with mitral valve disease generally are considered poor candidates for traditional open surgical replacement.
- Transcatheter mitral valve replacement (TMVR) can be performed with a balloon-expandable valve designed for transcatheter aortic valve replacement using a transseptal, transapical, or open transatrial approach.
- Although technically feasible, to date, TMVR in patients with severe MAC has been associated with high rates of procedural complications, 30-day mortality, and 1-year mortality.
- Important mechanisms of complications include left ventricular outflow tract (LVOT) obstruction and device malapposition with resultant regurgitation, migration, and embolization.
- The optimization of patient selection, mitral annular assessment, and predicted LVOT obstruction, in addition to device innovation, will be required to improve the short-term and long-term outcomes for this procedure.

INTRODUCTION

MAC is a fibrous, degenerative calcification of the mitral valve. It has been associated with endocarditis, coronary artery disease, valvular heart disease, and congestive heart failure.[1] Treatment of degenerative mitral valvular disease in the setting of MAC remains a challenge. Due to technical challenges and high perioperative mortality, patients with severe MAC associated with mitral valve disease are considered poor candidates for traditional surgery.[2] Transcatheter treatment of valvular disease has emerged as an alternative treatment option for patients with high surgical risk or intermediate surgical risk with severe symptomatic aortic stenosis.[3–7] This technology changed the therapeutic paradigm of aortic stenosis, leading to further expanded use of this technology to other etiologies, such as degenerative mitral valvular disease with MAC. The first reports of TMVR with the compassionate use of the balloon-expandable valves in this population showed successful results via surgical transapical or an open transatrial approach,[8–10] followed by a series of reports with completely percutaneous transfemoral (ie, transseptal) approach.[11–13] Despite these promising results, the safety and efficacy of TMVR in this population are unclear. Because transcatheter aortic valve replacement has specific complications, such as conduction

Disclosures: Dr R. Makkar has received grants from Edwards Lifesciences, United States and personal fees from St. Jude Medical, United States and Medtronic, United States. All other authors reported that they have no relationship relevant to the contents of this article to disclose.

Cedars-Sinai Smidt Heart Institute, 8700 Beverly Boulevard, Los Angeles, CA 90048, USA

* Corresponding author.

E-mail address: Raj.Makkar@cshs.org

Clinical vignette

A 90-year-old woman presented with severe symptomatic aortic stenosis. Her medical history included a stroke 15 years prior, with minimal residual impairment on the right hand, polymyalgia rheumatica, lumbar fracture, diabetes, and hypertension. She presented with exertional dyspnea and 1 episode of resting chest pain. Transthoracic echocardiogram revealed severe aortic stenosis with aortic valve area of 0.7 cm^2 and mean gradient of 40 mm Hg. Severe mitral annular calcification (MAC) also was noted. There was mild mitral stenosis and moderate-to-severe mitral regurgitation (Fig. 1A, B). The peak and mean transmitral gradients were 12 mm Hg and 6 mm Hg, respectively. Coronary angiography demonstrated no significant luminal obstruction. A heart team evaluation concluded that she was severely symptomatic with shortness of breath on minimal exertion but was also quite frail and thus not a surgical candidate for open, double-valve surgery. It was decided to treat her with transcatheter aortic valve replacement and to re-evaluate her mitral valve regurgitation thereafter. She underwent transfemoral transcatheter aortic valve replacement using a 23-mm Sapien 3 valve (Edwards Lifesciences, Irvine, United States) (see Fig. 1C). Postprocedure she had Mobitz type II atrioventricular block and received a permanent pacemaker. Her postprocedure course was uneventful and she subsequently was discharged to a skilled nursing facility for rehabilitation. At the time of discharge, she was found to have severe pulmonary hypertension associated with mitral regurgitation, which required further evaluation for potential transcatheter mitral valve replacement (TMVR) (see Fig. 1D). Her exertional dyspnea persisted postdischarge and eventually she was readmitted to the hospital for treatment of acute-on-chronic heart failure. Due to her multiple comorbidities, she was deemed extremely high risk for conventional surgical mitral valve replacement; she also was not a candidate for percutaneous edge-to-edge mitral valve repair due to the severe MAC. Therefore, TMVR for mitral regurgitation associated with severe MAC was considered an appropriate option. After extensive discussion with the patient's family, it was decided to proceed with TMVR with the Sapien 3. The family was explained the risks and benefits of the procedure, including a one-third risk of procedural death, a one-third chance of procedural success, and a one-third chance of successful procedure but without successful recovery due to extreme deconditioning and frailty. After reviewing the risks and benefits, the family and patient agreed to proceed with TMVR.

Anatomic evaluation demonstrated that she was at high risk for left ventricular outflow tract (LVOT) obstruction after TMVR for severe MAC. Multidetector CT (MDCT) showed extensive circumferential MAC. The mitral annulus dimensions included a trigon-to-trigon distance of 29.1 mm and a projected perimeter of 86 mm (Fig. 2A). Given the presence of extensive circumferential MAC, the 29-mm Sapien 3 valve was considered a potential transcatheter valve. To assess the risk of LVOT obstruction after the TMVR procedure, the authors simulated the procedure by embedding the virtual valve within the mitral annulus. The virtual valve with the same size of the 29-mm Sapien 3 was placed in the mitral annulus with an atrioventricular ratio of 30:70 (see Fig. 2B). After adjustment of the centerline of the aorta, the newly created LVOT (neo-LVOT) was simulated. By scrolling through the cross-sectional images of the neo-LVOT, the minimal neo-LVOT area was appreciated (see Fig. 2C, D). The minimal neo-LVOT area was 120 mm^2, suggesting extreme high risk for LVOT obstruction after TMVR. Therefore, it was decided to perform prophylactic alcohol septal ablation of the basal septum to decrease the risk of LVOT obstruction after TMVR.

The TMVR procedure was performed in the cardiac catheterization laboratory under general anesthesia and transesophageal echocardiogram (TEE). A 6-French guide catheter was used to engage the left coronary artery. A 0.014-in coronary guide wire was advanced into the first septal perforator of the left anterior descending artery. A 2.0-mm × 6-mm over-the-wire balloon was advanced into the proximal segment of the first septal perforator and inflated to 4 atm. Contrast was injected through the guide catheter as well as the over-the-wire balloon to ensure complete occlusion of the first septal perforator, and the territory perfused by the first septal perforator was confirmed with TEE. A total of 2 mL of dehydrated alcohol was injected through the over-the-wire balloon into the first septal perforator (Fig. 3A). A balloon-tipped temporary transvenous pacemaker was advanced through the femoral venous sheath and into the right ventricular apex. Then, the transseptal puncture was attempted under the fluoroscopy and TEE guidance. The sheath was slowly and carefully pulled back into the right atrium under TEE and fluoroscopic guidance, and the optimal site of septal puncture was identified. Then, the transseptal puncture was performed successfully at the midportion and slightly posterior aspect of the interatrial septum. The 8.5-French SL-1 (St. Jude Medical, United States) sheath was further advanced into the left atrium and patient was anticoagulated. A 0.32-mm guide wire was advanced into the left atrium through the SL-1 sheath and the sheath was removed. An 8.5-French medium-curve Agilis catheter was advanced into the left atrium and steered toward the mitral valve orifice, through which a 6-French pigtail catheter was advanced into the left atrium. A 6-French pigtail catheter was advanced into the left ventricle across the aortic valve (Fig. 3B). The pigtail catheter from the right femoral venous access then was advanced across the mitral valve into the left ventricle. A 0.035-in Confida guide wire was advanced into the left ventricle and the pigtail catheter was removed. A 16-French Sapien delivery sheath was inserted into the right femoral vein. A 12-mm × 4-mm Z-Med II balloon then was advanced across the interatrial septum, and an atrial septostomy was performed by inflating the balloon (see Fig. 3C). A 29-mm Sapien 3 Commander valve delivery system and the Sapien 3 valve was advanced through the right femoral venous Edwards sheath across the mitral valve annulus. The position of the transcatheter was confirmed with TEE and fluoroscopic landmarks for MAC. With rapid pacing at 180 beats per minute, the valve was deployed in the standard technique (see Fig. 3D). The patient was noted to experience persistent hypoxia after the valve deployment due to the right-to-left shunt across the iatrogenic atrial septal defect created by septal puncture and atrial septostomy. Therefore, the authors performed closure of the atrial septal defect with a 10-mm Amplatzer Septal Occluder. Postprocedural transthoracic echocardiogram showed acceptable hemodynamics, with a mean mitral valve gradient of 7 mm Hg. There was mild paravalvular regurgitation but no evidence of increased LVOT gradient. The total contrast volume used was 50 mL. Despite the successful TMVR procedure, the patient did develop uremic encephalopathy and was very lethargic postprocedure. She was started on multiple antibiotics for leukocytosis. One week after the TMVR procedure, she was found unresponsive, pulseless, and breathless. Cardiopulmonary resuscitation was performed but there was no spontaneous return of circulation.

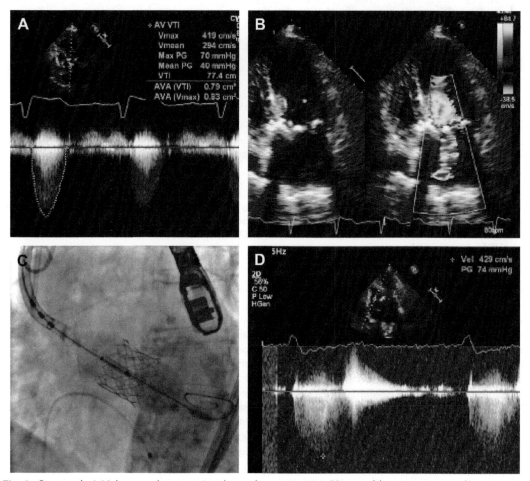

Fig. 1. Case study: initial transcatheter aortic valve replacement. (A) A 90-year-old woman presented severe aortic stenosis with mean gradient of 40 mm Hg and aortic valve area of 0.7 cm². (B) Moderate to severe mitral regurgitation also was noted. (C) A 23-mm Sapien 3 transcatheter valve was successfully implanted in the aortic position with transfemoral access. (D) Postprocedural transthoracic echocardiogram showed sustained severe pulmonary hypertension.

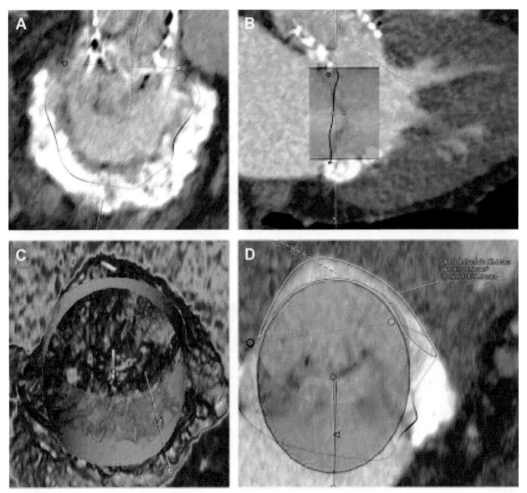

Fig. 2. Case study: assessment of mitral valve annulus and neo-LVOT area. (*A*) MDCT images of mitral annulus with circumferential severe MAC. (*B*) By embedding the virtual valve in the mitral annulus, TMVR was simulated. (*C*) 3-dimentional volume rendering image of the neo-LVOT. (*D*) After adjustment of the centerline of aorta, the neo-LVOT was estimated.

disturbances, paravalvular leak, and aortic root injury, TMVR poses unique and potentially fatal complication, such as LVOT obstruction. Understanding and prediction of these complications would help optimize the outcomes of TMVR in patients with severe MAC. This review article describes the procedural complications, clinical outcomes, and optimal patient selection of TMVR in patients with severe MAC.

LEFT VENTRICULAR OUTFLOW TRACT OBSTRUCTION

LVOT obstruction is the most catastrophic and unpredictable complication after TMVR. LVOT obstruction after surgical mitral valve procedures, such as mechanical valve replacement with the preservation of the anterior mitral

leaflet, has been reported,[14,15] particularly in patients with small ventricular cavity, such as those with mitral stenosis. Similarly, mitral valve-in-valve with the Sapien XT may result in a similar complication. TMVR in patients with previous mitral valve annuloplasty (valve-in-ring), however, may be at higher risk for LVOT obstruction because valve-in-ring procedures simulate surgical mitral valve replacement with preservation of anterior mitral leaflet. In this context, TMVR in patients with severe MAC may be at particularly high risk for LVOT obstruction because a majority of patients with severe MAC and mitral stenosis have a small ventricular cavity, and the anterior leaflet is preserved in its native state. Bapat and colleagues[16] first described the potential factors influencing LVOT obstruction after TMVR for patients with previous mitral

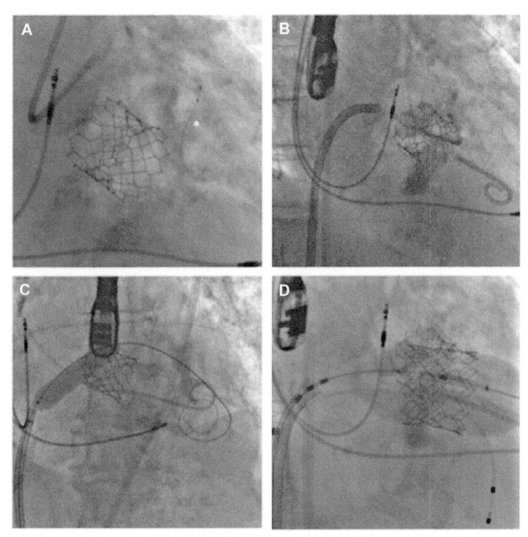

Fig. 3. Case study: TMVR. (*A*) Based on the MDCT assessment of risk for LVOT obstruction after TMVR, the patient underwent prophylactic alcohol septal ablation. (*B*) Septal puncture was successfully performed. (*C*) Strial septostomy was performed by inflating the balloon. (*D*) A 29-mm Sapien 3 valve was deployed in the mitral position via transseptal approach successfully.

bioprostheses (valve-in-valve) or mitral plasty rings. Through bench testing, the investigators concluded that the degree of LVOT obstruction was affected by the design of bioprostheses or rings, depth of implantation of the transcatheter valves, and the aortomitral angle. Given the challenges in estimating the risk of LVOT obstruction, Blanke and colleagues[17] proposed the concept of the neo-LVOT, defined by the newly created elongated outflow tract after transcatheter valve implantation. Wang and colleagues[18,19] proposed a CT-aided prediction model to identify patients at risk for LVOT obstruction. Nonetheless, these concepts still need to be validated with real-world data.

Yoon and colleagues[20] recently reported the predictors of LVOT obstruction after TMVR from an observational registry. The TMVR registry was created as an international, multicenter, observational study that enrolled consecutive patients undergoing TMVR for degenerated mitral bioprostheses, failed mitral annuloplasty rings, or severe MAC. Echocardiographic and procedural characteristics were recorded, and comprehensive MDCT assessment was performed at a dedicated core laboratory to identify the predictors of LVOT obstruction. Among 194 patients with preprocedural MDCT undergoing TMVR (valve-in-valve, 107 patients; valve-in-ring, 50 patients; and valve-in-MAC, 37 patients), LVOT obstruction was observed in 26 patients (13.4%). The rate of LVOT obstruction was the highest after valve-in-MAC (54.1%), followed by valve-in-ring (8.0%) and valve-in-valve (1.9%) (P<.001). Patients with LVOT obstruction had significantly higher procedural mortality compared with those without LVOT obstruction (34.6% vs 2.4%; P<.001). Receiver operating characteristic curve analysis showed that an estimated neo-LVOT area less than or equal to 1.7 cm^2 predicted LVOT obstruction, with sensitivity of 96.2% and specificity of 92.3% (Fig. 4). Although this study is limited by its inclusion of different patient subsets (ie, valve-in-valve, valve-in-ring, and valve-in-MAC), this information may help identify patients at high risk for LVOT obstruction after TMVR procedures.

PATIENT SELECTION

Given the high procedural mortality after LVOT obstruction after TMVR for valve-in-MAC

procedures, potential candidates should be evaluated for their risk of LVOT obstruction. As discussed previously, MDCT assessment of neo-LVOT area is the first step of the screening. Typically, mid to late systolic-phase MDCT images are used to reconstruct the neo-LVOT area with embedding of the virtual valve within the mitral position. The virtual valve with the same size of actual device is empirically simulated on the CT images with an atrioventricular ratio of 30:70. After manual correction of centerline, the neo-LVOT can be appreciated. The minimal neo-LVOT area is measured by planimetry by scrolling through the cross-sectional images of neo-LVOT. As discussed previously, a cutoff point of less than 1.7 cm^2 yielded high predictive value for LVOT obstruction. Therefore, from a practical perspective, patients with an estimated neo-LVOT area less than 2.0 cm^2 should be considered to be at high risk for LVOT obstruction after TMVR. Those patients with a high risk of LVOT obstruction may benefit from

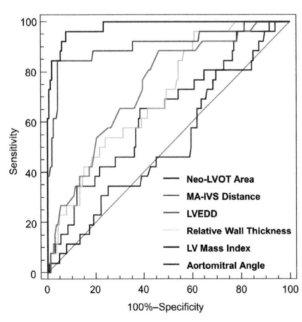

Fig. 4. (*Upper panel*) Receiver operating characteristic curves analyses for prediction of LVOT obstruction by MDCT and echocardiographic parameters. (*Lower panel*) Area under the curve, cut-off value, p value, sensitivity and specificity of each parameters. AUC, area under the curve; IVS, interventricular septum; LV, left ventricular; LVEDD, left ventricular end-diastolic diameter; MA, mitral annulus.

	AUC	Cutoff value	p value	Sensitivity	Specificity
Neo-LVOT Area	0.98	1.7	<.001	96.2	92.3
MA-IVS Distance	0.91	17.8	<.001	84.6	95.8
LVEDD	0.74	48	<.001	88.5	53.3
Relative Wall Thickness	0.70	0.38	.001	96.2	38.9
LV Mass Index	0.64	105	.02	65.4	61.1
Aortomitral Angle	0.51	–	0.92	46.2	41.1

prophylactic alcohol septal ablation or percutaneous laceration of the anterior mitral leaflet prior to valve implantation.

The mitral annular dimension should be also evaluated for TMVR in patients with severe MAC. Because a majority of the valve-in-MAC procedures have been done with balloon-expandable valves, the mitral annular dimension should be within the range of the available balloon-expandable devices. The presence of MAC, however, poses an issue for segmentation of the annulus with MDCT, because it can be difficult to correctly identify the boundary of the blood pool and calcified annular segments. Some calcifications are extremely dense and bulky, whereas a caseous pattern also is common. The device anchoring within the mitral annulus depends on the type and density of MAC. Unfortunately, there is no established methodology to assess the mitral annulus in patients with severe MAC. Future studies of valve-in-MAC need to propose a standardized approach to the measurement and segmentation of the mitral annulus, correlated with downstream procedural outcomes to provide robust guidance in this challenging area.

PROCEDURAL TECHNIQUE

The initial TMVR was performed for patients with degenerated mitral bioprostheses (valve-in-valve) via the transseptal and transatrial approach,[21] but difficulties in achieving a coaxial alignment of the transcatheter valve within the mitral bioprosthesis led to the transapical approach as a more feasible route thereafter.[22] Likewise, the initial successful reports of TMVR for severe MAC were via the transapical approach.[8,9] Advances in device technology with smaller profiles have enabled easier transseptal access. The decreased invasiveness of the transseptal compared with the transapical approach has been expected to result in superior outcomes. Nevertheless, none of previous studies demonstrated superiority of the transseptal approach over the transapical approach. Open transatrial TMVR with removal of the anterior mitral leaflet, which eliminates the challenges in predicting LVOT obstruction after TMVR, has showed promising results.[23] Given the early stage in the maturation process of TMVR for severe MAC, further investigation is needed for universal adoption of TMVR for patients with severe MAC.

For the transseptal approach, a modified technique can be used, in which the guide wire is externalized through a sheath percutaneously placed within the left ventricular apex. This modified technique can be used to improve coaxiality and support during valve deployment in cases of extreme valve leaflet calcification that potentially prevented coaxial positioning of the transcatheter valve. To decrease the risk of embolization, the transcatheter valve should be deployed in a conical shape and flared within the left ventricle.

OUTCOMES OF TRANSCATHETER MITRAL VALVE REPLACEMENT IN MITRAL ANNULAR CALCIFICATION

The initial report of Hasan and colleagues[8] demonstrated the feasibility of TMVR in patients with severe mitral stenosis associated with MAC. The 29-mm Sapien valves were implanted successfully via the transapical approach and provided acceptable hemodynamic outcomes (mean gradient of 7 mm Hg and no mitral regurgitation). Sinning and colleagues[9] also reported successful transapical TMVR for patients with severe MAC. Guerrero and colleagues[11] created the TMVR in MAC Global Registry to understand the safety and efficacy of TMVR in patients with severe MAC. Their initial report included 64 patients who underwent TMVR with compassionate use of a balloon-expandable transcatheter heart valve. The mean patient age was 73 years ± 13 years, 66% were female, and the mean Society of Thoracic Surgeons predicted operative mortality (STS PROM) was 14.4% ± 9.5%. The primary mitral valve pathology was stenosis in 93.5% of cases, whereas 6.5% had primarily mitral regurgitation. A transatrial delivery under direct visualization through an open surgical approach was used in a minority of cases (10 of 64 [15.6%]). Transapical and transseptal approaches were used in 28 cases (43.8%) and 26 cases (40.6%), respectively. Technical success according to the Mitral Valve Academic Research Consortium (MVARC) criteria (a procedure meeting all of the following: absence of procedural mortality; successful access, delivery, and retrieval of the device delivery system; successful deployment and correct positioning of the first intended device; and freedom from emergent surgery or reintervention related to the device or access) was achieved in 46 of 64 patients (72%), primarily limited by the need for a second valve implantation in 11 patients (17.2%). This was due to valve migration in 5 patients and regurgitation in 6 patients. Among those who required a second valve implantation due to mitral regurgitation, the mechanism was malposition that prevented adequate seal by the stent frame skirt in 5 patients. By the end of procedure, paravalvular regurgitation was mild or absent in all patients. There were 4 valve embolizations to the left atrium (6.25%), all of them during the index procedure. Six patients (9.3%) had LVOT obstruction with hemodynamic compromise after valve deployment. Among these patients, the average peak LVOT gradient was 72 mm Hg (range 39–100 mm Hg). Among those who had LVOT obstruction, only 1 patient survived after alcohol septal ablation. Periprocedural death occurred in 19 patients (29.7%; cardiovascular cause death in 12.5% and noncardiac in 17.2%). Of the 8 cardiovascular deaths, 2 were due to LVOT obstruction, 2 were secondary to left ventricular perforation, 2 were related to ischemic stroke, 1 was due to complete atrioventricular block, and 1 was due to acute myocardial infarction secondary to massive air embolism in the setting of guide wire–induced pulmonary vein perforation during a transapical procedure. Thirty-day follow-up echocardiographic data were obtained in 22 patients. The mean mitral valve gradient was 5.9 mm Hg $\pm$ 2.1 mm Hg ($P<.001$) with a mean mitral valve area of 2.3 cm^2 $\pm$ 0.8 cm^2 ($P<.001$). Eighteen patients (81.8%) had zero to trace mitral regurgitation and 4 (18.2%) had mild mitral regurgitation; no patients had moderate to severe mitral regurgitation. The average peak LVOT gradient was 15 mm Hg $\pm$ 17.8 mm Hg. Guerrero and colleagues concluded that TMVR with balloon-expandable valves for severe MAC was feasible in an extremely high-risk patient population. Technical success was achieved in most patients. Nonetheless, high rates of important complications and 30-day mortality were observed. LVOT obstruction defined as hemodynamic compromise occurred in 6 patients (9.3%) and 5 of these patients subsequently died. This highlights the impact of LVOT obstruction after TMVR on mortality and the importance of preprocedural screening for the risk of LVOT obstruction. Furthermore, high rates of second valve implantation (17.2%) and valve embolization to the left atrium (6.25%) emphasize the challenges in accurate measurement of the mitral annulus due to absence of evidence-based methodology for mitral annular assessment in patients with MAC.

Guerrero and colleagues[24] subsequently reported the 1-year outcomes of TMVR in severe MAC. A total of 116 patients were included. The mean patient age was 73 years $\pm$ 12 years, 68.1% were female, and the mean STS PROM was 15.3% $\pm$ 11.6%. Transseptal access was used in 40.5%, transapical access in 39.7%, and direct open transatrial access in 19.8%. Technical success according to MVARC criteria was achieved in 89 (76.7%) of the 116 patients, primarily limited by the need for implantation of a second valve. The hemodynamic results were acceptable, consistent with the initial report from this registry. LVOT obstruction with hemodynamic compromise occurred in 13 patients (11.2%). Of these patients, 5 were treated with medical management, 1 underwent kissing balloon aortic and mitral valvuloplasty, 1 underwent open surgery, and 6 were treated with alcohol septal ablation. Only 4 of the 13 patients with LVOT obstruction and hemodynamic compromise were discharged alive; all 4 had been treated with alcohol septal ablation. The 30-day all-cause mortality was 25% (cardiovascular, 13%, and noncardiovascular, 12%). During a median follow-up of 170 days (mean, 355 days; range, 50–1687 days), 57 patients died (1-year all-cause mortality, 53.7%; cardiovascular, 23.5%; and noncardiovascular, 30.2%) (Fig. 5). The investigators concluded that most patients who survived the 30-day postprocedural period remained alive at 1 year. Patient age, New York Heart Association (NYHA) functional class, transapical or transseptal versus transatrial access, LVOT obstruction, valve embolization, and conversion to open surgery were identified as predictors of 1-year mortality on univariate Cox regression analysis. LVOT obstruction was a strong predictor of 30-day and 1-year mortality (hazard ratio 3.16; 95% CI, 1.19–8.36; $P = .02$; and hazard ratio, 3.56; 95% CI, 1.81–7.01; $P<.001$, respectively). Most patients had sustained improvement of symptoms. At 1 year, 28 of the 39 patients with data available had NYHA functional class I or class II symptoms (71.8%). Echocardiographic follow-up at 1 year was available in 34 (70.8%) of 49 patients alive. There was a significant improvement in mean mitral valve gradient (5.8 $\pm$ 2.2 mm Hg; $P<.001$ vs baseline) and mitral valve area (1.9 $\pm$ 0.5 cm^2; $P<.011$ vs baseline). Twenty-four (75%) patients had no to trace mitral regurgitation, 7 (21.9%) patients had mild mitral regurgitation, and 1 patient (3.1%) had severe paravalvular regurgitation. The average peak LVOT gradient was 7.3 mm Hg $\pm$ 10.8 mm Hg ($P = .16$ vs baseline). Compared with the first half of the patients in the registry, the second half tended to have lower rates of 30-day mortality (19% vs 31%; $P = .07$) and second valve implantation (19% vs 10.3%; $P = .09$), consistent with an improvement in outcomes with increasing operator experience. Nonetheless, these findings should be cautiously interpreted.

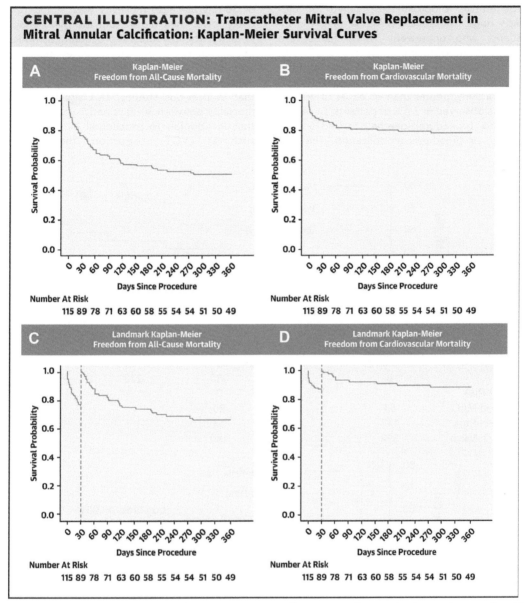

CENTRAL ILLUSTRATION: Transcatheter Mitral Valve Replacement in Mitral Annular Calcification: Kaplan-Meier Survival Curves

A Kaplan-Meier Freedom from All-Cause Mortality

B Kaplan-Meier Freedom from Cardiovascular Mortality

C Landmark Kaplan-Meier Freedom from All-Cause Mortality

D Landmark Kaplan-Meier Freedom from Cardiovascular Mortality

Number At Risk
115 89 78 71 63 60 58 55 54 54 51 50 49

Fig. 5. Kaplan-Meier survival curves of TMVR in MAC. (*A*) All-cause mortality. (*B*) Cardiovascular mortality. (*C*) Landmark analysis of all-cause mortality TMVR after 30 days. (*D*) Landmark analysis of cardiovascular mortality after 30 days. (*Reprinted from* Guerrero M, Urena M, Himbert D, et al. 1-Year outcomes of transcatheter mitral valve replacement in patients with severe mitral annular calcification. J Am Coll Cardiol 2018;71(17):1841–53; with permission from Elsevier.)

As Ramzy and colleagues[25] commented, Guerrero and colleagues[29] expanded the registry from the initial report, but the additional 2 years of experience did not show improved outcomes of TMVR in severe MAC. In particular, the rate of LVOT obstruction remained as high as 11.2% and did not decrease in the second half of their 1-year report. Given the limitations of the registry, it is possible that this rate was even under-reported. This implies a significant learning curve for clinicians with respect to the technical aspect but also for patient selection. Because LVOT obstruction was a major determinant of 1-year survival, it is clear that all potential candidates for TMVR in patients with severe MAC should be evaluated for the risk of LVOT obstruction by an evidence-based methodology.

Urena and colleagues[26] reported their single-center 7-year experience of TMVR for degenerative bioprostheses, failed annuloplasty rings, and severe MAC. Among the 27 patients who underwent TMVR for severe MAC, the rate of technical success was 77.7%, mainly limited by a high rate of second valve implantation (22.2%). LVOT obstruction, defined as a gradient greater than or equal to 50 mm Hg, was observed in 7.4% of patients, but there were no procedural deaths, conversions to surgery, or prosthesis embolization. The rate of 30-day all-cause mortality was 11.1%, relatively lower than those from the MAC Global Registry. The low rates of procedural complications from this experienced center may have contributed to this result. Nonetheless, 1-year all-cause mortality was 44.4%, comparable to that of previous studies. This significant late mortality between 30-days and 1-year suggests that in addition to procedural complications, such as LVOT obstruction, the baseline

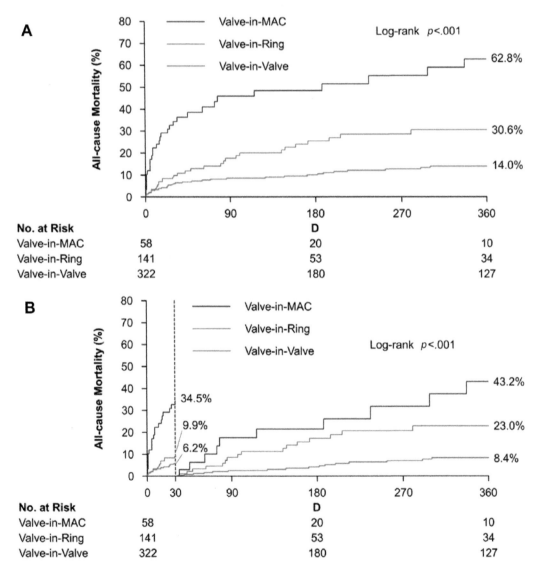

Fig. 6. All-cause mortality according to TMVR procedure. (A) Time-to-event curves for all-cause mortality of patients undergoing mitral valve-in-valve (green line), valve-in-ring (blue line), and valve-in-MAC (red line) are shown. (B) Time-to-event curves for all-cause mortality with landmark analyses (0–30 days and 30–360 days) showed increased early mortality (0–30 days) but also late mortality (30–360 days) after valve-in-MAC compared with valve-in-ring and valve-in-valve. (From Yoon SH, Whisenant BK, Bleiziffer S, et al. Outcomes of transcatheter mitral valve replacement for degenerated bioprostheses, failed annuloplasty rings, and mitral annular calcification. Eur Heart J 2019;40(5):441–51; with permission.)

comorbidities associated with calcific mitral valve disease likely affected the long-term mortality. The 2-year all-cause mortality was higher in patients with valve-in-MAC than those with valve-in-valve or valve-in-ring (58.4% vs 29.4% vs 24.5%; log-rank $P = .038$). The presence of MAC was reported as an indicator of atherosclerosis burden and has been associated with an increased risk of late cardiovascular and overall mortality.[27]

The TMVR registry recently reported the outcomes of TMVR for patients with severe MAC and compared them to those with degenerated bioprostheses and failed annuloplasty rings. A total of 521 patients underwent TMVR (valve-in-valve, 322 patients; valve-in-ring, 141 patients; and valve-in-MAC, 58 patients). The mean STS PROM in the valve-in-MAC group was 10.1% ± 6.9%. Transseptal and transapical access were used in 53.4% and 44.8% of patients, respectively. Balloon-expandable Sapien valves (Sapien, Sapien XT, and Sapien 3) were used in 81.0% of patients. In line with previous reports, high rates of procedural complications were observed. Conversion to surgery and valve embolization were observed in 8.6% and 6.9%, respectively. Implantation of a second valve was required in 5.2%. LVOT obstruction according to the MVARC criteria (increment in mean gradient ≥10 mm Hg from baseline) was observed in 23 patients (39.7%). Technical success was achieved in 36 patients (62.1%). Reintervention was performed in 13 patients (22.4%): alcohol septal ablation in 7 patients; atrial septal defect closure in 6; and surgical mitral valve replacement in 1. Postprocedural echocardiography demonstrated favorable results with a mean mitral valve gradient of 5.4 mm Hg ± 3.1 mm Hg and a mean mitral valve area of 2.6 cm^2 ± 1.1 cm^2. There was a fairly high rate, however, of residual moderate or higher mitral regurgitation at postprocedure (13.8%) and at 30 days (13.2%). All-cause mortality at 30 days and 1 year were 34.5% and 62.8%, respectively, significantly higher than that observed in the valve-in-ring (9.9% and 30.6%) and valve-in-valve groups (6.2% and 14.0%) (Fig. 6). The strikingly high rate of LVOT obstruction in the TMVR registry may be attributable to the following: (1) inconsistent assessment of risk for LVOT obstruction with imaging modalities and (2) variable definitions of LVOT obstruction between the studies. A comprehensive analysis of mitral valve and left ventricular anatomy to predict LVOT obstruction is essential for optimal patient selection. Furthermore, prophylactic alcohol septal ablation and laceration of mitral anterior leaflet have recently emerged as options to prevent TMVR-associated LVOT obstruction and hold promise for mitigating this catastrophic complication.[28,29]

SUMMARY

Outcomes data to date for TMVR in severe MAC demonstrate that this procedure is associated with high rates of serious complications and, in turn, substantial short-term and midterm mortality. TMVR with current available valve technology is technically feasible but further advancements are required to improve outcomes, including device innovation and patient selection using an evidence-based risk assessment for the potential of LVOT obstruction.

REFERENCES

1. D'Cruz I, Panetta F, Cohen H, et al. Submitral calcification or sclerosis in elderly patients: M mode and two dimensional echocardiography in "Mitral anulus calcification". Am J Cardiol 1979;44:31–8.

2. Papadopoulos N, Dietrich M, Christodoulou T, et al. Midterm survival after decalcification of the mitral annulus. Ann Thorac Surg 2009;87: 1143–7.

3. Leon MB, Smith CR, Mack M, et al. Transcatheter aortic-valve implantation for aortic stenosis in patients who cannot undergo surgery. N Engl J Med 2010;363:1597–607.

4. Smith CR, Leon MB, Mack MJ, et al, PARTNER Trial Investigators. Transcatheter versus surgical aortic-valve replacement in high-risk patients. N Engl J Med 2011;364:2187–98.

5. Adams DH, Popma JJ, Reardon MJ, et al, Investigators USCC. Transcatheter aortic-valve replacement with a self-expanding prosthesis. N Engl J Med 2014;370:1790–8.

6. Leon MB, Smith CR, Mack MJ, et al, PARTNER 2 Investigators. Transcatheter or surgical aortic-valve replacement in intermediate-risk patients. N Engl J Med 2016;374:1609–20.

7. Reardon MJ, Van Mieghem NM, Popma JJ, et al, SURTAVI Investigators. Surgical or transcatheter aortic-valve replacement in intermediate-risk patients. N Engl J Med 2017;376:1321–31.

8. Hasan R, Mahadevan VS, Schneider H, et al. First in human transapical implantation of an inverted transcatheter aortic valve prosthesis to treat native mitral valve stenosis. Circulation 2013;128:e74–6.

9. Sinning JM, Mellert F, Schiller W, et al. Transcatheter mitral valve replacement using a balloon-expandable prosthesis in a patient with calcified native mitral valve stenosis. Eur Heart J 2013;34: 2609.

10. Wilbring M, Alexiou K, Tugtekin SM, et al. Pushing the limits-further evolutions of transcatheter valve procedures in the mitral position, including valve-in-valve, valve-in-ring, and valve-in-native-ring. J Thorac Cardiovasc Surg 2014;147:210–9.

11. Guerrero M, Greenbaum A, O'Neill W. First in human percutaneous implantation of a balloon expandable transcatheter heart valve in a severely stenosed native mitral valve. Catheter Cardiovasc Interv 2014;83:E287–91.

12. Fassa AA, Himbert D, Brochet E, et al. Transseptal transcatheter mitral valve implantation for severely calcified mitral stenosis. JACC Cardiovasc Interv 2014;7:696–7.

13. Himbert D, Bouleti C, Iung B, et al. Transcatheter valve replacement in patients with severe mitral valve disease and annular calcification. J Am Coll Cardiol 2014;64:2557–8.

14. Rietman G, Vandermaaten J, Douglas Y, et al. Echocardiographic diagnosis of left ventricular outflow tract obstruction after mitral valve replacement with subvalvular preservation. Eur J Cardiothorac Surg 2002;22:825–7.

15. Wu Q, Zhang L, Zhu R. Obstruction of left ventricular outflow tract after mechanical mitral valve replacement. Ann Thorac Surg 2008;85:1789–91.

16. Bapat V, Pirone F, Kapetanakis S, et al. Factors influencing left ventricular outflow tract obstruction following a mitral valve-in-valve or valve-in-ring procedure, part 1. Catheter Cardiovasc Interv 2015;86:747–60.

17. Blanke P, Naoum C, Dvir D, et al. Predicting LVOT obstruction in transcatheter mitral valve implantation: concept of the Neo-LVOT. JACC Cardiovasc Imaging 2017;10:482–5.

18. Wang DD, Eng M, Greenbaum A, et al. Predicting LVOT obstruction after TMVR. JACC Cardiovasc Imaging 2016;9:1349–52.

19. Wang DD, Eng MH, Greenbaum AB, et al. Validating a prediction modeling tool for left ventricular outflow tract (LVOT) obstruction after transcatheter mitral valve replacement (TMVR). Catheter Cardiovasc Interv 2018;92:379–87.

20. Yoon SH, Bleiziffer S, Latib A, et al. Predictors of left ventricular outflow tract obstruction after transcatheter mitral valve replacement. JACC Cardiovasc Interv 2019;12:182–93.

21. Webb JG, Wood DA, Ye J, et al. Transcatheter valve-in-valve implantation for failed bioprosthetic heart valves. Circulation 2010;121:1848–57.

22. Cheung A, Webb JG, Barbanti M, et al. 5-year experience with transcatheter transapical mitral valve-in-valve implantation for bioprosthetic valve dysfunction. J Am Coll Cardiol 2013;61:1759–66.

23. Russell HM, Guerrero ME, Salinger MH, et al. Open atrial transcatheter mitral valve replacement in patients with mitral annular calcification. J Am Coll Cardiol 2018;72:1437–48.

24. Guerrero M, Urena M, Himbert D, et al. 1-year outcomes of transcatheter mitral valve replacement in patients with severe mitral annular calcification. J Am Coll Cardiol 2018;71:1841–53.

25. Ramzy D, Chung J, Trento A. Transcatheter mitral valve replacement for severe mitral annular calcification: is it ready for prime time? J Am Coll Cardiol 2018;71:1854–6.

26. Urena M, Brochet E, Lecomte M, et al. Clinical and haemodynamic outcomes of balloon-expandable transcatheter mitral valve implantation: a 7-year experience. Eur Heart J 2018;39:2679–89.

27. Fox CS, Vasan RS, Parise H, et al. Mitral annular calcification predicts cardiovascular morbidity and mortality: the Framingham Heart Study. Circulation 2003;107:1492–6.

28. Babaliaros VC, Greenbaum AB, Khan JM, et al. Intentional percutaneous laceration of the anterior mitral leaflet to prevent outflow obstruction during transcatheter mitral valve replacement: first-in-human experience. JACC Cardiovasc Interv 2017;10:798–809.

29. Guerrero M, Wang DD, Himbert D, et al. Short-term results of alcohol septal ablation as a bail-out strategy to treat severe left ventricular outflow tract obstruction after transcatheter mitral valve replacement in patients with severe mitral annular calcification. Catheter Cardiovasc Interv 2017;90:1220–6.

Surgical Transatrial Implantation of Transcatheter Heart Valves in Severe Mitral Annular Calcification

Mohammad Kassar, MD[a], Omar K. Khalique, MD[b],
Thomas Pilgrim, MD[a], David Reineke, MD[c],
Thierry Carrel, MD[c], Stephan Windecker, MD[a],
Isaac George, MD[d], Fabien Praz, MD[a],*

KEYWORDS

- Mitral regurgitation • Mitral stenosis • Mitral valve • Mitral annular calcification
- Transcatheter mitral valve • Left ventricular outflow tract obstruction

KEY POINTS

- Surgical transatrial mitral valve implantation of a transcatheter heart valve is a feasible hybrid treatment option in patients with mitral valve disease related to mitral annular calcification.
- The transatrial access offers several advantages, in particular a very low risk of left ventricular outflow tract obstruction as a result of systematic resection of the anterior mitral valve leaflet.
- Patients not suitable for transfemoral/transseptal or transapical access due to increased risk of valve embolization or left ventricular outflow tract obstruction can be safely treated via the transatrial approach.
- Early reports show favorable hemodynamic results, although overall mortality in these highly morbid patients remains high, and therefore careful patient selection is required.

INTRODUCTION

The treatment of patients requiring mitral valve (MV) replacement due to advanced MV stenosis and/or regurgitation associated with severe annular calcification is a challenge for the cardiac surgeon. First, affected patients tend to be older and have multiple comorbidities.[1] Second, the inability to pass sutures through the calcified

Conflicts of interest: O.K. Khalique has received speaker fees from Edwards Lifescience; T. Pilgrim has received research grants to the institution from Edwards Lifesciences, Symetis/Boston Scientific, and Biotronik, and speaker fees from Boston Scientific and Biotronik; T. Carrel has received financial support from Xeltis AG, Zurich, Switzerland. S. Windecker has received research grants to the institution from Abbott, Amgen, Boston Scientific, Biotronik, and St. Jude Medical. I. George has received consulting fees for Edwards Lifesciences, Medtronic, and Boston Scientific. F. Praz has served as a consultant for Edwards Lifesciences. The remaining authors declare no conflict of interest.
[a] Department of Cardiology, Bern University Hospital, Freiburgstrasse 4, Bern 3011, Switzerland; [b] Structural Heart and Valve Center, Division of Cardiology, New York-Presbyterian Hospital-Columbia University Medical Center, 630 West 168th Street, New York City, NY 10032, USA; [c] Department of Cardiovascular Surgery, Bern University Hospital, Freiburgstrasse 4, Bern 3011, Switzerland; [d] Department of Cardiothoracic Surgery, New York-Presbyterian Hospital-Columbia University Medical Center, 630 West 168th Street, New York City, NY 10032, USA
* Corresponding author. Bern University Hospital, Freiburgstrasse 4, Bern 3011, Switzerland.
E-mail address: fabien.praz@insel.ch

mitral annulus (MA) precludes MV repair and complicates MV replacement.

Various modified surgical techniques, for example, selective segmental decalcification, atrial sliding plasties, anterior leaflet transposition, and autologous or xenograft patch plasty have been proposed.[2–4] However, these methods may lead to prolonged duration of cardiopulmonary bypass and are associated with complications like patient-prosthesis mismatch due to the use of an undersized valve, bleeding, paravalvular leak, injury to the left circumflex artery, rupture of the atrioventricular grove, and debris embolization. Many patients with mitral annular calcification (MAC) are turned down for MV surgery because of these limitations. Open transatrial implantation of a transcatheter heart valve (THV) has been proposed as a possible alternative in selected patients. Compared with the transseptal approach, it has the advantage to minimize the risk of left ventricular outflow tract obstruction (LVOTO) as a result of systematic resection of the anterior MV leaflet. Since its first description by Carrel and colleagues[5] in 2012, the procedure has evolved owing to technical modifications and improved imaging methods.

EPIDEMIOLOGY OF MITRAL ANNULAR CALCIFICATION

MAC of any severity is present in 8% to 15% of the general population, predominantly affecting elderly patients.[6–9] Among candidates for transcatheter aortic valve replacement (TAVR) and patients with chronic renal failure, its frequency is as high as 49% and 42%, respectively.[10,11] In addition to age, other predictors of MAC include female gender, osteoporosis, obesity, and the usual cardiovascular risk factors.[6,12] Genetic hypertriglyceridemia has been more specifically linked to MAC in a recent population-based study including 5651 individuals.[13] MAC is a marker of higher cardiovascular morbidity and mortality, probably because of its frequent association with atherosclerosis, as well as with MV stenosis and regurgitation.[1] Furthermore, severe calcification of the MA has been associated with conduction abnormalities after TAVR, highlighting the close location to the conduction system and the importance of aorto-mitral interactions in patients with multivalvular disease.[10]

The degenerative process observed in MAC generally involves the posterior aspect of the annulus in a semilunar fashion and less frequently extends to the anterior portions. It may be circumferential and occasionally involve the aorto-mitral curtain. Later in the course of the disease, direct calcification of the valve leaflets may be observed and result in MV disease. However, only a minority of patients with MAC develop relevant MV disease. Mitral stenosis in combination with MAC is present in 0.2% of patients undergoing transthoracic echocardiography,[14] whereas MAC is observed in 11.7% of the patients with severe mitral regurgitation.[15]

PATIENT SELECTION AND TRANSCATHETER HEART VALVE SIZING
Mitral Annulus Sizing

Diagnosis, staging and anatomic assessment of MV disease includes conventional transthoracic and transesophageal echocardiography (TEE). The use of 2-dimensional echocardiography is limited because of foreshortening and geometric assumptions. Due to high spatial resolution and overall usability, multi-sliced computed tomography (CT) has emerged as the primary imaging tool for MV annulus sizing. Three-dimensional (3D)-TEE may be considered as an adjunctive method and has shown excellent agreement with CT measurements.[16] Different imaging methods may be used, including multiplanar reconstruction (**Fig. 1**A, B) or cubic spline interpolation during end-diastole (70%–80%). The calcified annulus is delineated following the inner border of the calcium. The aorto-mitral curtain is systematically excluded in the presence of an anterior calcium rim. Due to irregularities of the calcification patterns, the perimeter may overestimate the actual dimensions of the annulus. Thus, valve selection using aortic sizing charts should be based on valve area, area-derived perimeter, or averaged diameter (defined as the average of the maximal and minimal diameter).

Direct visualization and balloon sizing during the procedure are essential for final selection of the prosthesis (**Fig. 1**C), especially in case of disagreement between noninvasive sizing methods.

Assessment of the Risk of Left Ventricular Outflow Tract Obstruction

Valve implantation in the mitral position is associated with a risk of LVOTO that is influenced by several device-related and anatomic factors, including the length and mobility of the anterior MV leaflet; the dimensions of the left ventricular cavity; the presence of an intraventricular septum bulge; aorto-mitral angulation; and implant protrusion into the left ventricular outflow tract (LVOT) (**Box 1**).

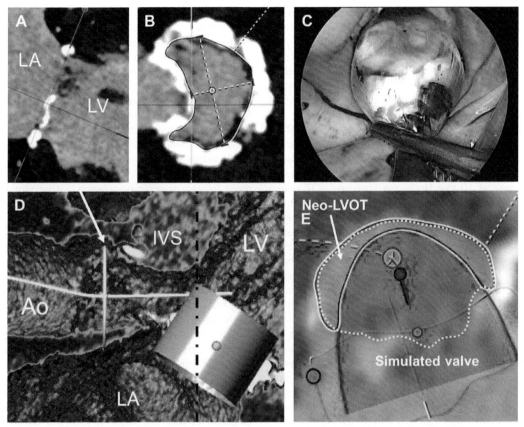

Fig. 1. MA sizing and prediction of the Neo-LVOT. (A) Example of CT measurement of the MA using multiplanar reconstruction. Biplanar adjustment at the level of the calcified annulus is performed. (B) The inner borders are traced. (C) Intraoperative balloon sizing. The balloon should fit snugly to the annulus borders using nominal volume. The corresponding next larger valve size is typically chosen. (D) Valve simulation in the reconstructed 3D anatomy mimicking the final valve implantation target. The arrow indicates the aortic annular plane and the interrupted line the plane of maximal valve protrusion used for measurement of the LVOT and neo-LVOT. (E) Determination of the neo-LVOT area. The yellow interrupted line represents the native LVOT (for didactic purpose both lines do not exactly overlap). Ao, aorta; LA, left atrium; LV, left ventricle; IVS, interventricular septum.

These parameters coalesce to build the "neo-LVOT"[17] that may significantly differ from the native LVOT with respect to its 3D shape and cross-sectional area. Although an insignificant increase of the blood velocity across the neo-LVOT is frequently recorded after percutaneous MV replacement, insufficient dimensions of the neo-LVOT may result in immediate obstruction, which represents a potentially lethal complication.

To anticipate clinically significant LVOTO, valve simulation has been proposed and a corresponding protocol implemented into current imaging software (eg, 3Mensio Structural Heart Mitral Workflow version 8.1 Pie Medical Imaging, Maastricht, the Netherlands).

During preprocedural planning of a valve implantation in mitral position, the virtual valve model is placed at the level of the MV annulus in a position that mimics the final implantation target (typically 30% atrial and 70% ventricular for the transfemoral/transseptal and transapical approach). Adjustment is performed through 3D rotation of the model (Fig. 1D). The neo-LVOT and the total LVOT areas are measured at the

---

Box 1
Factors associated with risk of left ventricular outflow tract obstruction

Length and mobility of the anterior mitral valve leaflet

Dimensions of the left ventricular cavity

Presence of an intraventricular septum bulge

Aorto-mitral angulation

Implant protrusion into the left ventricular outflow tract

level of maximal stent frame protrusion during systole (typically 30%–40% phase) (Fig. 1E). The most predictive time point in systole has not yet been determined; however, late-systole likely overestimates the risk of LVOTO as all of the stroke volume has been ejected from the ventricle. Based on prior experience in transcatheter valve-in-valve cases, a neo-LVOT area of 250 mm^2 or more should have low risk of LVOTO even using the transfemoral/transseptal or transapical access. An absolute neo-LVOT area less than 189.4 mm^2 has been shown to predict an increase of 10 mm Hg in the invasive LVOT peak gradient after transcatheter MV replacement in 38 patients undergoing various MV interventions.[18] Although it has not been systematically studied, individualized cutoffs considering the relative LVOT reduction may apply, rather than absolute neo-LVOT area. Patients with a neo-LVOT area considered high risk for obstruction should be considered for the open transatrial approach.

After resection of the anterior MV leaflet, a THV can be safely implanted even in patients at high risk for LVOTO. The stent frame protruding into the LVOT is left uncovered and allows for blood flow. In the 26 patients of the largest series published so far,[19] the mean anticipated neo-LVOT area was 135 ± 64 mm^2 (range, 42–268 mm^2) corresponding to a mean relative LVOT reduction (defined as [LVOT area − neo-LVOT area/LVOT area] × 100) of 61% ± 15%, indicating high risk of LVOTO. Despite the small anticipated neo-LVOT, only 1 patient who received a clearly oversized THV experienced clinically relevant postprocedural elevation of the mean transvalvular aortic gradient (30 mm Hg). This is likely explained by protruding fabric skirt of the THV obstructing the LVOT, despite resection of the anterior native valve leaflet (so called skirt neo-LVOT[20]).

Computer modeling[21] and 3D printing[22] have been proposed as complementary strategies for preprocedural planning.

ADVANTAGES AND DISADVANTAGES OF THE SURGICAL TRANSATRIAL ACCESS

Thanks to direct visualization and access to the MV apparatus, the transatrial approach offers several advantages, including direct balloon sizing for final THV selection; controlled valve positioning and deployment; a low risk of LVOTO after resection of the anterior leaflet (leaving the stent frame protruding into the LVOT uncovered); a low risk of significant residual paravalvular leak and valve embolization

using dedicated surgical techniques; and the possibility to perform a concomitant surgical myomectomy if necessary.

Patient screening for dedicated trials of transcatheter MV replacement has demonstrated that a high proportion (approximately two-thirds) of the patients with relevant MAC are not suitable for the transfemoral/transseptal or transapical approach due to the increased risk of LVOTO. Thus, the development of interventional or surgical techniques to minimize this risk may broaden the access to transcatheter MV replacement for this specific population. Other strategies in candidates with anticipated high risk of LVOTO include intentional laceration of the anterior MV leaflet (LAMPOON),[23] as well as preemptive or emergent alcohol septal ablation.[24,25]

There are several other advantages of the transatrial implantation technique in patients with MAC. The application of anchoring sutures to the atrial wall or leaflet tissue minimizes the risk of embolization and may enable the treatment of patients with large annular areas (up to 800 mm^2) who would not qualify for other approaches. Stability of the valve can be manually verified before access closure. In rare instances, the subvalvular apparatus may be calcified as well and interact with the delivery system during valve positioning and deployment via the transfemoral/transseptal or transapical approach. Selective resection of calcified chordae and/or papillary muscles is also possible when using the transatrial technique. Furthermore, the transatrial approach using median sternotomy allows for concomitant valve surgery of the aortic and tricuspid valve, as well as surgical revascularization, if required.

On the other hand, disadvantages include greater invasiveness potentially resulting in higher periprocedural mortality, as well as a requirement for cardiac arrest and cardiopulmonary bypass.

IMPLANTATION TECHNIQUES

Early Experience and Procedural Steps

The first open transatrial THV implantation into a MAC was performed in 2012 at Bern University Hospital, Switzerland, in a patient initially scheduled for conventional MV replacement due to mixed MV disease.[5] Following a median sternotomy and standard cardioplegic arrest, the MV was exposed through a left atriotomy. Even after partial resection of the anterior and posterior MV leaflets, the orifice was deemed too small for the placement of a surgical bioprosthesis of appropriate size, and thus, the decision was made to implant a THV Edwards SAPIEN XT (Edwards Lifesciences, Irvine, CA) valve under direct visualization. The MV orifice was sized using a 24-mm balloon and a 26-mm valve was selected. The SAPIEN XT valve was crimped on the Edwards Ascendra transapical system. The assembly was then advanced into the left ventricle and the valve slowly deployed into the calcified annulus. Circularization of the elliptical MA was observed. Manual dislodgement of the valve was attempted to confirm stable position. Four sutures were placed into the atrial tissue surrounding the annulus to further prevent embolization. A paravalvular leak detected by saline probe was closed with an additional stich. The final mean transmitral gradient was 2 mm Hg with mild paravalvular leak and the patient was discharged after 8 days. During further experience, paravalvular leakage sometimes associated with hemolysis was identified as potential complication negatively influencing outcomes, justifying the development of dedicated preventive strategies.[26]

Strategies to Prevent Paravalvular Leakage

In patients with MAC, paravalvular leak is typically related to the irregular contours of the calcium deposits around the MA preventing tight apposition of the stent frame. The adoption of second-generation THVs featuring a skirt around the inflow, for example, the Lotus[27] or the SAPIEN 3 valve,[19,26] may improve sealing. Sewing of a felt strip around the valve inflow in combination with the placement of several sutures along the leaflet tissue before valve implantation have been proposed as additional measures to prevent paravalvular leak.[19,28,29]

Preparation consists of securing a 0.75-cm to 1.0-cm soft felt strip to the base of the THV stent frame (**Fig. 2**A) and subsequent crimping on the transapical (Ascendra/Certitude) delivery system

in the usual fashion. Ideally, the commissures of the THV should be marked, as they generate the highest flow limitation and should not be placed into the LVOT during implantation, but rather oriented toward the postulated location of the trigones. Concurrently, pledgeted sutures are placed along the annulus through leaflet tissue. Excessive manipulation or debridement of the MA should be avoided to prevent debris embolization. The valve is then slowly deployed under visual control by the first operator (**Fig. 2**B), ensuring correct location of the covered inflow at the annular level. After the sutures have been tightened, postdilatation, using additional volume if appropriate, is of crucial importance to optimize valve expansion and apposition (**Fig. 2**C). This step may be associated with a small risk of annular rupture.

Another method, the "extended collar technique," has been described. A circular collar, consisting of either Teflon or pericardial patch material, is prepared and sutured to the inflow of the stent frame mimicking the design of some of the dedicated transcatheter MV replacement devices. Annular sutures to left atrial tissue are then fixed to the inner border of the collar, adjacent to the stented valve and tied down to ensure correct positioning at the annulus level. Additional atrial sutures may be placed in regions with incomplete contact to the atrial wall.

Alternative Options for Surgical Access

Although most of the reported cases were performed via a median sternotomy, the use of a right thoracotomy has been described.[30] This approach has the advantage to reduce the invasiveness of the procedure, in particular for patients presenting with chronic lung disease. When anterolateral thoracotomy is performed, cardiopulmonary bypass is obtained via femoral cannulation. Only a few on-pump beating heart procedures have been reported. In such cases,

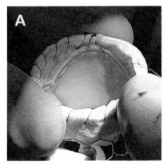 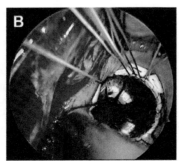 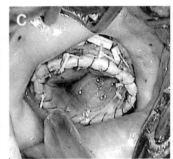

Fig. 2. Strategies to prevent paravalvular leakage. (*A*) Sewing of a felt strip at the inflow of the Edwards Sapien 3 valve. (*B*) Valve implantation after placement of pledgeted sutures along the annulus. (*C*) Final result after postdilatation with good sealing confirmed by saline probe.

fluoroscopy supports correct positioning of the valve into the MAC.[26]

Outcomes Data

In the early experience, 2 small series reported the outcomes of 4[31] and 6 patients.[26] The risk of LVOTO in the absence of resection of the anterior leaflet was demonstrated in the first study. Partial transaortic resection allowed for normalization of the LVOT gradients. In another patient, surgical septal myectomy was performed to prevent obstruction. The second study described the risks of paravalvular leak and valve embolization that may be associated with the early surgical technique. This, together with associated comorbidities, translated into a high mortality of 50% at 30 days.

In the largest study published to date, 26 patients were treated using the previously described modified technique consisting of felt strip and pledgeted sutures placement.[19] This was found to almost eliminate the risks of paravalvular leak and valve embolization resulting in high procedural success according to the Mitral Valve Academic Research Consortium (MVARC) criteria[32] (100%). The mean transmitral gradient decreased from 10 ± 5 mm Hg to 4 ± 2 mm Hg ($P<.001$) along with functional improvement in most patients discharged alive. Mortality at 30 days remained high (27%), mainly because of complications related to the learning curve (eg, embolization due to excessive manipulations and debridement of the calcified annulus) as well as patient comorbidities. Kidney failure and presence of multivalvular disease were associated with adverse outcomes.

A more recent series reported favorable outcomes in 8 patients treated at a single center.[29] Procedural and device success according to MVARC criteria were both 100%. One patient developed hemolysis related to mild paravalvular leak 6 months after the procedure that was successfully addressed by percutaneous device closure.

Careful patient selection as well as the development of hybrid strategies (eg, concomitant or staged TAVR) may further improve the applicability of this novel surgical technique.

SUMMARY

Surgical transatrial THV implantation may be chosen for patients with MAC who are not amenable to the transapical or transfemoral/transseptal approach due to unfavorable anatomy. The main advantage of this approach is to enable resection of the anterior MV leaflet

and thus minimize the risk of LVOTO. The 2 complications associated with most periprocedural deaths observed in the early experience of transatrial THV implantation for MAC are paravalvular leak and valve embolization. Refined surgical techniques reduce the occurrence of this adverse event. Mortality remains high in these patients with multiple comorbidity, and therefore careful patient selection is necessary. Further investigations are required to understand better which patients are optimal candidates based on procedural timing, medical history, and anatomy.

REFERENCES

1. Fox CS, Vasan RS, Parise H, et al. Mitral annular calcification predicts cardiovascular morbidity and mortality: the Framingham Heart Study. Circulation 2003;107(11):1492–6.
2. Carpentier AF, Pellerin M, Fuzellier JF, et al. Extensive calcification of the mitral valve anulus: pathology and surgical management. J Thorac Cardiovasc Surg 1996;111(4):718–29 [discussion: 29–30].
3. Feindel CM, Tufail Z, David TE, et al. Mitral valve surgery in patients with extensive calcification of the mitral annulus. J Thorac Cardiovasc Surg 2003;126(3):777–82.
4. Carrel TP, Weber A. Selective, segmental decalcification: a safe alternative to extensive debridement of a severely calcified annulus during repair of mitral regurgitation. Interact Cardiovasc Thorac Surg 2016;23(4):665–7.
5. Carrel T, Wenaweser P, Reineke S, et al. Worldwide first surgical implantation of a transcatheter valved stent in mitral position. Cardiovasc Med 2012;15(6): 202–5.
6. Kanjanauthai S, Nasir K, Katz R, et al. Relationships of mitral annular calcification to cardiovascular risk factors: the Multi-Ethnic Study of Atherosclerosis (MESA). Atherosclerosis 2010;213(2):558–62.
7. Allison MA, Cheung P, Criqui MH, et al. Mitral and aortic annular calcification are highly associated with systemic calcified atherosclerosis. Circulation 2006;113(6):861–6.
8. Fertman MH, Wolff L. Calcification of the mitral valve. Am Heart J 1946;31:580–9.
9. Foley PW, Hamaad A, El-Gendi H, et al. Incidental cardiac findings on computed tomography imaging of the thorax. BMC Res Notes 2010;3:326.
10. Abramowitz Y, Kazuno Y, Chakravarty T, et al. Concomitant mitral annular calcification and severe aortic stenosis: prevalence, characteristics and outcome following transcatheter aortic valve replacement. Eur Heart J 2017;38(16):1194–203.

11. Asselbergs FW, Mozaffarian D, Katz R, et al. Association of renal function with cardiac calcifications in older adults: the cardiovascular health study. Nephrol Dial Transplant 2009;24(3):834–40.

12. Davutoglu V, Yilmaz M, Soydinc S, et al. Mitral annular calcification is associated with osteoporosis in women. Am Heart J 2004;147(6):1113–6.

13. Afshar M, Luk K, Do R, et al, CHARGE Extracoronary Calcium Working Group. Association of triglyceride-related genetic variants with mitral annular calcification. J Am Coll Cardiol 2017; 69(24):2941–8.

14. Akram MR, Chan T, McAuliffe S, et al. Non-rheumatic annular mitral stenosis: prevalence and characteristics. Eur J Echocardiogr 2009;10(1):103–5.

15. Movahed MR, Saito Y, Ahmadi-Kashani M, et al. Mitral annulus calcification is associated with valvular and cardiac structural abnormalities. Cardiovasc Ultrasound 2007;5:14.

16. Mak GJ, Blanke P, Ong K, et al. Three-dimensional echocardiography compared with computed tomography to determine mitral annulus size before transcatheter mitral valve implantation. Circ Cardiovasc Imaging 2016;9(6) [pii:e004176].

17. Blanke P, Naoum C, Dvir D, et al. Predicting LVOT obstruction in transcatheter mitral valve implantation: concept of the neo-LVOT. JACC Cardiovasc Imaging 2017;10(4):482–5.

18. Wang DD, Eng MH, Greenbaum AB, et al. Validating a prediction modeling tool for left ventricular outflow tract (LVOT) obstruction after transcatheter mitral valve replacement (TMVR). Catheter Cardiovasc Interv 2018;92(2):379–87.

19. Praz F, Khalique OK, Lee R, et al. Transatrial implantation of a transcatheter heart valve for severe mitral annular calcification. J Thorac Cardiovasc Surg 2018;156(1):132–42.

20. Khan JM, Rogers T, Babaliaros VC, et al. Predicting left ventricular outflow tract obstruction despite anterior mitral leaflet resection: the "Skirt NeoLVOT". JACC Cardiovasc Imaging 2018;11(9):1356–9.

21. de Jaegere P, Rajani R, Prendergast B, et al. Patient-specific computer modeling for the planning of transcatheter mitral valve replacement. J Am Coll Cardiol 2018;72(8):956–8.

22. Bagur R, Cheung A, Chu MWA, et al. 3-dimensional-printed model for planning transcatheter mitral valve replacement. JACC Cardiovasc Interv 2018;11(8):812–3.

23. Babaliaros VC, Greenbaum AB, Khan JM, et al. Intentional percutaneous laceration of the anterior mitral leaflet to prevent outflow obstruction during transcatheter mitral valve replacement: first-in-human experience. JACC Cardiovasc Interv 2017; 10(8):798–809.

24. Guerrero M, Wang DD, Himbert D, et al. Short-term results of alcohol septal ablation as a bail-out strategy to treat severe left ventricular outflow tract obstruction after transcatheter mitral valve replacement in patients with severe mitral annular calcification. Catheter Cardiovasc Interv 2017;90(7):1220–6.

25. Sayah N, Urena M, Brochet E, et al. Alcohol septal ablation preceding transcatheter valve implantation to prevent left ventricular outflow tract obstruction. EuroIntervention 2017;13(17):2012–3.

26. El Sabbagh A, Eleid MF, Foley TA, et al. Direct transatrial implantation of balloon-expandable valve for mitral stenosis with severe annular calcifications: early experience and lessons learned. Eur J Cardiothorac Surg 2018;53(1):162–9.

27. Ghosh-Dastidar M, Bapat V. Transcatheter valve implantation in mitral annular calcification during open surgery: extended collar technique. Ann Thorac Surg 2017;104(3):e303–5.

28. Lee R, Fukuhara S, George I, et al. Mitral valve replacement with a transcatheter valve in the setting of severe mitral annular calcification. J Thorac Cardiovasc Surg 2016;151(3):e47–9.

29. Russell HM, Guerrero ME, Salinger MH, et al. Open atrial transcatheter mitral valve replacement in patients with mitral annular calcification. J Am Coll Cardiol 2018;72(13):1437–48.

30. Nissen AP, Lamelas J, George I, et al. Minimally invasive transatrial mitral valve replacement in mitral annular calcification. Ann Cardiothorac Surg 2018;7(6):827–9.

31. Langhammer B, Huber C, Windecker S, et al. Surgical antegrade transcatheter mitral valve implantation for symptomatic mitral valve disease and heavily calcified annulus. Eur J Cardiothorac Surg 2017;51(2):382–4.

32. Stone GW, Adams DH, Abraham WT, et al, Mitral Valve Academic Research Consortium (MVARC). Clinical trial design principles and endpoint definitions for transcatheter mitral valve repair and replacement: part 2: endpoint definitions: a consensus document from the mitral valve academic research consortium. J Am Coll Cardiol 2015;66(3):308–21.

Moving?

Make sure your subscription moves with you!

To notify us of your new address, find your **Clinics Account Number** (located on your mailing label above your name), and contact customer service at:

Email: journalscustomerservice-usa@elsevier.com

800-654-2452 (subscribers in the U.S. & Canada)
314-447-8871 (subscribers outside of the U.S. & Canada)

Fax number: 314-447-8029

Elsevier Health Sciences Division
Subscription Customer Service
3251 Riverport Lane
Maryland Heights, MO 63043

*To ensure uninterrupted delivery of your subscription, please notify us at least 4 weeks in advance of move.